ABC of
Urology

Third Edition

ABC series

An outstanding collection of resources – written by specialists for non-specialists

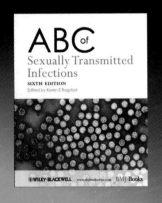

ABC of Sexually Transmitted Infections
SIXTH EDITION
Edited by Karen E Rogstad

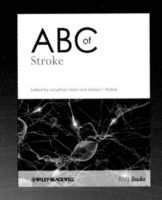

ABC of Stroke
Edited by Jonathan Mant and Marion F Walker

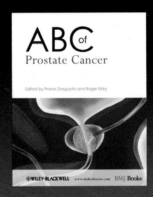

ABC of Prostate Cancer
Edited by Prokar Dasgupta and Roger Kirby

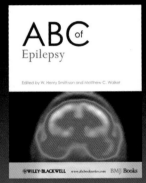

ABC of Epilepsy
Edited by W. Henry Smithson and Matthew C. Walker

The *ABC* series contains a wealth of indispensable resources for GPs, GP registrars, junior doctors, doctors in training and all those in primary care

▶ **Now fully revised and updated**
▶ **Highly illustrated, informative and a practical source of knowledge**
▶ **An easy-to-use resource, covering the symptoms, investigations, treatment and management of conditions presenting in day-to-day practice and patient support**
▶ **Full colour photographs and illustrations aid diagnosis and patient understanding of a condition**

For more information on all books in the *ABC* series, including links to further information, references and links to the latest official guidelines, please visit:

www.abcbookseries.com

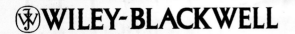

WILEY-BLACKWELL

BMJ|Books

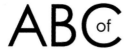

ABC of

Urology

Third Edition

EDITED BY

Chris Dawson

Consultant Urological Surgeon
Peterborough and Stamford NHS Foundation Trust, Peterborough, UK

Janine M. Nethercliffe

Consultant Urological Surgeon
Peterborough and Stamford NHS Foundation Trust, Peterborough, UK

WILEY-BLACKWELL

A John Wiley & Sons, Ltd., Publication

BMJ|Books

This edition first published 2012 © 2012 by John Wiley & Sons, Ltd.

BMJ Books is an imprint of BMJ Publishing Group Limited, used under licence by Blackwell Publishing which was acquired by John Wiley & Sons in February 2007. Blackwell's publishing programme has been merged with Wiley's global Scientific, Technical and Medical business to form Wiley-Blackwell.

Registered office: John Wiley & Sons, Ltd, The Atrium, Southern Gate, Chichester, West Sussex, PO19 8SQ, UK

Editorial offices: 9600 Garsington Road, Oxford, OX4 2DQ, UK
The Atrium, Southern Gate, Chichester, West Sussex, PO19 8SQ, UK
111 River Street, Hoboken, NJ 07030-5774, USA

For details of our global editorial offices, for customer services and for information about how to apply for permission to reuse the copyright material in this book please see our website at www.wiley.com/wiley-blackwell.

The right of the author to be identified as the author of this work has been asserted in accordance with the UK Copyright, Designs and Patents Act 1988.

Library of Congress Cataloging-in-Publication Data
ABC of Urology / edited by Chris Dawson, Janine M. Nethercliffe, – 3rd ed.
    p. ; cm. – (ABC series)
  Includes bibliographical references and index.
  ISBN 978-0-470-65717-1 (pbk.)
  I. Dawson, Chris, MB BS. II. Nethercliffe, Janine M. III. Series: ABC series (Malden, Mass.)
  [DNLM: 1. Urologic Diseases – diagnosis. 2. Urologic Diseases – therapy. 3. Genital Diseases, Male – diagnosis. 4. Genital Diseases, Male – therapy. WJ 140]
  616.6 – dc23
                                                                            2011044209

A catalogue record for this book is available from the British Library.

Wiley also publishes its books in a variety of electronic formats. Some content that appears in print may not be available in electronic books.

Set in 9.25/12 Minion by Laserwords Private Limited, Chennai, India
Printed and bound in Malaysia by Vivar Printing Sdn Bhd

1 2012

Contents

Contributors

James Allan
Consultant Urologist
St Edmonds Hospital, Bury St Edmonds, Suffolk, UK

Jonathan Aning
Specialist Registrar
Department of Urology, Derriford Hospital, Plymouth, UK

Simon R.J. Bott
Consultant Urologist
Frimley Park Hospital, Surrey, UK

Richard Cetti
Specialist Registrar
Department of Urology, St Richard's Hospital, Chichester, West Sussex, UK

Nim Christopher
Consultant Urologist
Institute of Urology, University College London Hospital,
London, UK

Peter Cuckow
Consultant Paediatric Urologist
Great Ormond Street Hospital, London, UK

William J.G. Finch
Specialty Registrar in Urology
Peterborough and Stamford Hospitals NHS Foundation Trust,
Peterborough, UK

Simon J. Freeman
Consultant Radiologist
Derriford Hospital, Plymouth, UK

Tamsin Greenwell
Consultant Urological Surgeon
Honorary Senior Lecturer, University College London Hospitals,
London, UK

Helen Hegarty
Consultant Urological Surgeon
Southend University Hospital NHS Foundation Trust, Essex, UK

Richard Johnston
Senior Fellow in Urology
Addenbrooke's Hospital, Cambridge, UK

Farooq A. Khan
Consultant Urologist
Luton & Dunstable Foundation NHS Trust, Luton, UK

Stephen E.M. Langley
Professor of Urology
The Royal Surrey County Hospital and St Luke's Cancer Centre,
Surrey, UK

Danish Mazhar
Consultant Medical Oncologist
Oncology Centre, Addenbrooke's Hospital, Cambridge, UK

Esther McLarty
Consultant Urological Surgeon
Department of Urology, Derriford Hospital, Plymouth, UK

Janine M. Nethercliffe
Consultant Urological Surgeon
Peterborough and Stamford NHS Foundation Trust,
Peterborough, UK

Pippa Sangster
Urology Specialist Registrar
Kingston Hospital NHS Trust, Kingston Upon Thames, Surrey, UK

Majid Shabbir
Senior Andrology Fellow
Department of Andrology, Institute of Urology, University College
London Hospital, London, UK

Nimish Shah
Consultant Urologist
Addenbrooke's Hospital, Cambridge, UK

Deborah Skennerton
Consultant Urologist
Epsom Hospital, Surrey, UK

Daniel Swallow
Urology ST4 Trainee
Luton & Dunstable Hospital NHS Foundation Trust,
Luton, UK

Alan Thompson
Consultant Urological Surgeon
Royal Marsden Hospital NHS Foundation Trust,
Surrey, UK

Suzie Venn
Consultant Urological Surgeon
Western Sussex Hospitals Trust and Queen Alexandra Hospital,
Portsmouth, UK

Anne Y. Warren
Consultant Histopathologist
Cambridge University Hospitals NHS Foundation Trust
Associate Lecturer
Cambridge University, Cambridge, UK

Jessica Wrigley
Oncology Specialist Registrar
Department of Oncology, Addenbrooke's Hospital,
Cambridge, UK

Preface

Since the first edition of the ABC of Urology was written 15 years ago there have been fundamental changes in the way that Urology is practiced. It seems to us that things change ever more quickly and the last 5 years has seen particularly rapid change.

Such change has led to the production of the 3rd edition of the ABC of Urology.

The remit of the book remains the same as when it was originally conceived; to inform and educate trainees in surgery, nursing and staff in other disciplines about the latest developments in Urology. The book remains a valuable introduction to the field of Urology and will be useful for surgeons in training for the MRCS.

To this extent we are very pleased to have co-opted leading Urology specialists to write chapters for this book.

All of the chapters have been revised and there have been major additions, particularly in laparoscopy, and in the addition of separate chapters on Management of Haematuria, and Penile Cancer. All of the cancer chapters have been extensively re-written and provide a current and comprehensive guide to management.

We are indebted to the staff of Wiley; without their help and patience this book would not have been written.

Chris Dawson and Janine M. Nethercliffe

Dedication

This book is dedicated to Rachel, James, and Claire, who provide so much love and support.

Chris Dawson

CHAPTER 1

Assessment of the Urological Patient

Deborah Skennerton

OVERVIEW
- A careful history and examination is required to elicit the correct symptoms and signs
- The majority of the urinary system is not amenable to clinical examination and further investigations are normally required

---

Assessment of the urological patient starts with a careful history of the presenting complaint and where appropriate assessment of the impact of these symptoms on quality of life. Clinical examination and appropriate investigation help to make a diagnosis.

Urological symptoms

- Pain
- Haematuria
- Storage LUTS
- Voiding LUTS
- Urinary incontinence
- Sexual dysfunction

Pain

Genitourinary tract pain is usually associated with obstruction or inflammation. Tumours rarely cause pain unless causing obstruction or invading surrounding nerves.

Renal pain

Renal pain is located in the costovertebral angle and may radiate anteriorly across the abdomen to the groin and genitalia. It is caused by distension of the renal capsule due to obstruction or inflammation. Pain is typically colicky in obstruction as ureteric peristalsis increases renal pelvic pressure, but steady in inflammation. Musculoskeletal disorders affecting T10–12 may also cause pain in the renal area but the pain is positional.

Bladder pain

Bladder pain is caused by overdistension due to acute retention or inflammatory conditions. Slowly progressive obstruction causing chronic retention is painless despite residuals of over 1 litre. Inflammatory conditions of the bladder cause intermittent suprapubic pain, typically worse when the bladder is full. Cystitis can also cause sharp, suprapubic pain at the end of micturition or, in men, penile tip pain, termed strangury. Strangury is also seen in renal colic as a stone traverses the intramural part of the ureter.

Prostatic pain

Prostatic pain is due to inflammation causing distension of the prostate capsule. It is poorly localised to the lower abdomen, perineum or rectum, and frequently associated with irritative voiding symptoms.

Testicular pain

Testicular pain may be due to scrotal pathology or referred pain. Inflammatory conditions of the scrotal contents or torsion cause acute pain. Chronic pain is usually due to non-inflammatory conditions such as varicocele or hydrocele. However, renal colic can also cause pain referred to the scrotum.

Haematuria

Haematuria may be painful or painless, visible or non-visible (found on urine dipstick or microscopy). Visible haematuria increases the likelihood of finding underlying pathology.

Causes of haematuria

- Infection/inflammation
- Malignancy
- Stones
- Benign prostatic enlargement
- Trauma

Consumption of beetroot can also result in discoloured urine so haematuria should be confirmed by microscopy.

Lower urinary tract symptoms (LUTS)

Storage symptoms

- Frequency
- Nocturia
- Urgency +/- incontinence
- Dysuria

Adults normally void up to 7 times a day. Voiding once a night may be considered normal. Urinary frequency is either due to a reduced bladder capacity or due to excess urine production. Completing a 3-day bladder diary will enable objective assessment of bladder capacity and frequency. Urge incontinence is particularly bothersome as it often results in large volume urine loss and is exacerbated by reduced mobility in the elderly population. Frequency may also be due to infection.

Voiding symptoms

- Hesitancy
- Slow flow
- Intermittent flow
- Straining

Patients reliably describe needing to wait before voiding (hesitancy) or straining to achieve urine flow. They are often unaware of a decrease in their urine flow until severely restricted such that the flow no longer shoots forward but trickles down towards their toes. A sensation of incomplete bladder emptying correlates poorly with measurements of residual volume.

Incontinence

Careful questioning will usually determine the circumstances of urine loss. Patients' response to urine loss will depend on their fastidiousness but may be influenced by race and culture. Men will often dribble a small amount of urine from the meatus after voiding – post-micturition dribble. This can be eased by 'milking' the urethra. An idea of volume loss will be gained by enquiring about the number of incontinence pads used.

Types of urinary incontinence

- Stress
- Urge
- Continuous
- Overflow

Stress incontinence results from increasing intra-abdominal pressure above urethral resistance. Urine loss is in small amounts and may affect both sexes but is more common in women with a weak pelvic floor following childbirth. Urge incontinence results in

larger volume loss and needs to be distinguished from stress leakage as it may indicate underlying bladder pathology. Continuous urine leakage in women is seen in vesicovaginal fistulae. Overflow incontinence is seen with a chronically distended bladder. Urine leakage usually occurs at night resulting in bed-wetting.

Sexual dysfunction

Patients often find discussing their sexual dysfunction difficult due to embarrassment but also because they lack the language to explain their symptoms. The presence of early morning erections or erection with masturbation rules out organic impotence. Retrograde ejaculation is common after prostate surgery and with the use of alpha-blockers for LUTS. Premature ejaculation is subjective and usually psychogenic.

Symptoms of sexual dysfunction

- Erectile dysfunction
- Loss of libido
- Disorders of ejaculation
- Penile curvature

Examination

Although it is tempting to skip examination in favour of radiological investigation, along with a careful history, examination is a key component in diagnostic evaluation.

Abdomen

Much of the renal tract lies deep to the examining hand and abnormalities will only be detected on imaging. However, in a thin patient it may be possible to see a grossly distended bladder although in obese patients this may be difficult to detect even with percussion.

External genitalia

The penis and scrotum lie easily accessible between the thighs. The foreskin should be retracted to examine the glans and meatus. The meatus should be gently parted to ensure there is no stenosis. Palpation of the penile shaft will reveal any Peyronie's plaques, typically found dorsally.

Scrotal examination should be carried out gently when an inflammatory condition or torsion is suspected. Each testis and epididymis should be examined for tenderness or masses. A firm or hard area in a testis should be considered a malignant tumour until proven otherwise. Masses in the epididymis are almost always benign.

Vaginal examination

With the patient's legs abducted, the introitus should be inspected for atrophic changes or inflammatory lesions, which may cause dysuria. The patient should be asked to perform a Valsalva manoeuvre and be examined for prolapse. Stress incontinence may be elicited with coughing, but it should be remembered that patients may not leak when supine and will often empty their bladder before being examined to prevent embarrassment. Failure to elicit leakage does not mean patients do not leak. Bimanual examination should be performed in lower urinary tract symptoms to detect an abnormality of the cervix or pelvic mass.

Rectal examination

Rectal examination is undignified and uncomfortable but carried out carefully should not be painful unless there is anal pathology or prostatic inflammation present. Patients should be examined in the left lateral position with the knees brought up to meet the elbows. Anal tone and perianal sensation can be assessed. A well-lubricated index finger can be slowly inserted into the anal canal and the prostate palpated through the anterior wall of the rectum. Only a small proportion of the two prostate lobes with their midline sulcus can be felt. Thus assessment of prostate size is notoriously inaccurate. The prostate should be non-tender and smooth, with no hard, craggy areas. The finger should sweep around the rest of the assessable rectum before removing to exclude an incidental rectal tumour.

Investigation

Urine dipstick

Dipstick testing (Figure 1.1) is quick and simple, and should be performed in all patients with urinary symptoms. Glycosuria may be the first sign of diabetes in a patient complaining of LUTS. Dipstick testing is not diagnostic of infection and if suspected a midstream sample should be sent for culture before empirical antibiotics are commenced. Non-visible haematuria (dipstick or microscopic) may be intermittent and should prompt referral for further investigation.

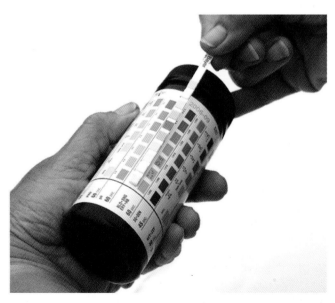

Figure 1.1 Urine dipsticks can be read manually, as shown, or using an electronic reader.

Urine culture

Culture of a midstream sample is the only way to identify patients whose symptoms truly result from infection. Positive urine cultures in the absence of white cells probably represent contaminated samples. Sterile pyuria may be seen when a sample is taken after commencement of antibiotics or early after treatment of a urinary tract infection (UTI), but may also be seen in stones and tumours, and rarely in tuberculosis (TB). Sterile pyuria is defined as >10 white cells per mm^3 of urine.

Urine cytology

The diagnostic yield of cytology is poor except in high-grade tumours and does not replace diagnostic cystoscopy.

Biochemistry

Most hospitals now report estimated glomerular flitration rate (eGFR) based on plasma creatinine. However, creatinine is inaccurate for early renal loss and does not rise until more that half of nephron function is lost. Prostate specific antigen (PSA) testing should be offered to men with lower urinary tract symptoms after appropriate discussion about its value and limitations.

Ultrasound

Ultrasound scanning (USS) is a safe, painless and low-cost diagnostic imaging technique in adults, as well as in children. Accurate interpretation of real time images by the operator is paramount as static images rarely convey all the information.

USS is particularly useful in renal impairment and where contrast is contra-indicated. Renal size can be determined along with cortical thickness, scarring and anatomical abnormalities. Dilatation of the collecting system (hydronephrosis) may point to distal obstruction although the cause may be difficult to see with USS. Solid renal masses can be differentiated from cystic lesions. Small renal stones may be difficult to visualise, whilst it is also possible to miss a stone filling the renal pelvis. Imaging the kidney can be difficult in obese patients.

A full bladder is easily seen with transabdominal ultrasound and may detect bladder tumours or stones. USS can also be used to assess bladder capacity and post-micturition urine volume.

Transrectal USS of the prostate can be used to measure prostate volume and to look for anatomical abnormalities in infertility. Prostate biopsy and minimally invasive treatments for prostate cancer are carried out under USS guidance.

Scrotal USS (Figure 1.2) is very accurate at detecting testicular tumours. It is also useful in inflammatory conditions or tense hydroceles where clinical examination may be difficult. This should not be relied upon in suspected testicular torsion. Many men with scrotal pain are reassured by a normal USS scan.

Cystoscopy

Cystoscopy is the mainstay of investigation of bladder symptoms. Flexible cystoscopy is routinely used in the setting of the one-stop haematuria clinic but rigid cystoscopy under a general anaesthetic makes up a large proportion of the operative workload of a urology department.

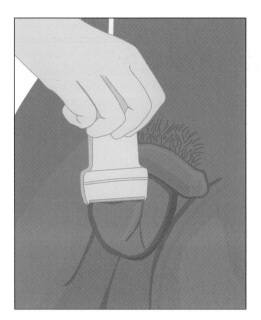

Figure 1.2 Scrotal ultrasound.

Urodynamic investigation of bladder function

A flow rate (Figure 1.3) is the basic urodynamic investigation. It is non-invasive and simply requires the patient to empty their full bladder into the machine for an objective assessment of flow. This is usually combined with measurement of residual urine with a bladder scanner. A slow flow may indicate obstruction but may also be seen in a hypocontractile bladder.

Where diagnostic concern remains pressure/flow urodynamics can be performed where a small pressure transducer is inserted into the bladder to measure bladder pressure when the patient voids.

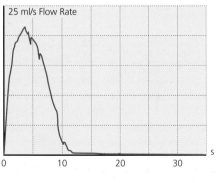

Results of UROFLOWMETRY

Voiding Time	T100	11	s
Flow Time	TQ	11	s
Time to Max Flow	TQmax	3	s
Max Flow Rate	Qmax	21.5	ml/s
Average Flow Rate	Qave	12.6	ml/s
Voided Volume	Vcomp	144	ml

Figure 1.3 Flow-rate.

This is usually combined with filling cystometry where the bladder pressure is measured whilst being artificially filled. This is useful for investigation of incontinence or irritative LUTS.

In complex cases the bladder may be filled with contrast medium during urodynamics to look at the bladder neck and sphincter mechanism (videourodynamics).

Radiological investigation

Plain radiography (KUB) and intravenous urography (IVU)

Ninety per cent of renal calculi are radio-opaque, but a KUB on its own is of limited value in renal colic as small ureteric stones cannot be differentiated from non-urinary calcifications. Following contrast the level of obstruction will reveal the offending stone. IVU is also used in the investigation of haematuria.

Computerised tomography (CT)

In many departments, non-contrast CT has replaced the IVU as the investigation of choice in renal colic or complex stone disease.

Contrast CT is used for characterisation of renal masses, assessment of renal trauma and as a second-line investigation of haematuria. Sophisticated reconstruction of images aids planning of complex surgery.

Magnetic resonance imaging (MRI)

The primary role of MRI in urological investigation is in staging of prostate cancer. MRI is also used to differentiate adrenal adenomas from malignant tumours and to delineate the anatomy of urethral diverticula in women.

Nuclear imaging

The handling characteristics of different radiopharmaceuticals give information on both renal function and anatomy.

Static isotope renography with DMSA (dimercaptosuccinic acid) will identify renal scarring and gives split renal function. Dynamic renography with MAG3 (mercapto acetyl triglycine) is used to identify obstruction of the kidneys and will also give split renal function.

Isotope bone scans are used in uro-oncology to identify bone metastases.

Further reading

Smith's General Urology. Emil A Tanagho and Jack W McAninch. McGraw-Hill Medical, 2008.

Campbell's Urology, 8th ed. Patrick Walsh, Alan B Retik, E Darracott Vaughn Jr et al, Saunders, 2002.

BAUS Guidelines. http://www.baus.org.uk/NR/rdonlyres/469ADC2B-62BA-4714-B432-53FB35E13803/0/haematuria_consensus_guidelines_July_2008.pdf.

CHAPTER 2

Guidelines for the Management of Haematuria

Daniel Swallow

Introduction

Haematuria is the presence of blood in the urine. It has urological and non-urological causes, both benign and malignant. It can also be classified into non-visible and visible haematuria. Visible haematuria means that there is sufficient blood in the urine to colour it either red or brown. Non-visible haematuria is subdivided into symptomatic and non-symptomatic types and was hitherto referred to as microscopic haematuria.

Haematuria is a very common reason for referrals to urology departments, often as an urgent problem.

Detection of non-visible haematuria in primary care is the initial step in a series of investigations, and is usually done using urine dipsticks. These grade non-visible haematuria from 'trace' to '3+'. '1+' or more is considered to be a positive reading (trace should be considered negative). There can be occasional false positive results caused by hypochlorite solutions, oxidising agents or bacterial

activity (the dipstick uses oxidation of an organic peroxide by haemoglobin as its mechanism).

The causes of haematuria

The causes of haematuria can be grouped anatomically or aetiologically. Anatomically the source of the haematuria could be the upper tract (kidneys or ureters) or the lower urinary tract (bladder, prostate or urethra). Investigations are specifically targeted at these constituent parts: ultrasound and x-ray for the upper tract, and cystoscopy for the lower urinary tract. Aetiologically the possible causes include tumours, stones or infections in any of the constituent parts of the urinary tract (see Box 2.1). Drug abuse with ketamine is becoming an increasingly common cause of haematuria in younger patients. In either case, patients with haematuria will almost invariably require further investigation.

Box 2.1

Urological causes of haematuria:
- Cancer – most commonly transitional cell carcinoma (bladder, kidney, urethra, ureter) or renal cell carcinoma (kidney)
- Stones – kidney, ureter, bladder
- Urinary tract infection [UTI] (cystitis, pyelonephritis etc.)
- Trauma (including instrumentation or catheterisation)
- Benign prostatic hypertrophy or prostate cancer causing prostatic bleeds

The management of patients with haematuria

The following groups of patients require investigation:

- Any episode of visible haematuria
- Any episode of *symptomatic* non-visible haematuria (in the absence of urinary tract infections (UTI) or other transient causes) – Box 2.2
- *Persistent asymptomatic* non-visible haematuria (in the absence of UTI or other transient causes), i.e. 2 or 3 positive dipstick readings

ABC of Urology, Third Edition.
Edited by Chris Dawson and Janine M. Nethercliffe.
© 2012 John Wiley & Sons, Ltd. Published 2012 by John Wiley & Sons, Ltd.

The investigation of haematuria

All patients with visible haematuria (any age), those with symptomatic non-visible haematuria (again, any age), and those with asymptomatic non-visible haematuria if aged 40 or over should be referred to a one-stop haematuria clinic.

The investigations shown in Figure 2.1 should be preceded by baseline tests performed in primary care, including estimated glomerular filtration rate (eGFR) or plasma creatinine and urine dipstick testing to exclude urinary tract infection and to determine the presence or absence of proteinuria. The prostate specific antigen (PSA) should be measured in men, after appropriate counselling because prostate cancer can present with haematuria. There are disadvantages of measuring PSA and these are shown in Box 2.3. Blood pressure should also be measured as this may indicate a nephrological cause.

The history taking should determine the chronology of the haematuria, whether it was painful, whether there is a history of anticoagulation, whether there was associated dysuria, and should include a general picture of any other urological symptoms.

The physical examination should include a brief general examination looking for performance status and weight loss, followed by an abdominal examination, specifically looking for flank masses. Rectal examination must be performed in men to assess the prostate.

All patients will then undergo an ultrasound and x-ray of the kidneys and ureters and bladder (KUB), followed by cystoscopy, usually performed under local anaesthesia. If clinically appropriate, patients will also undergo urine cytology testing, or PSA testing if this has not already been done (see Box 2.3).

If the ultrasound scan shows a mass lesion in the kidneys then an urgent CT urogram is required (Figure 2.2).

Flexible cystoscopy

Flexible cystoscopy is the gold-standard investigation for the lower urinary tract. Modern flexible cystoscopes have a fibre-optic light source mounted at the end of a fine, flexible telescope. This is either connected to a monitor, or the surgeon must look directly into

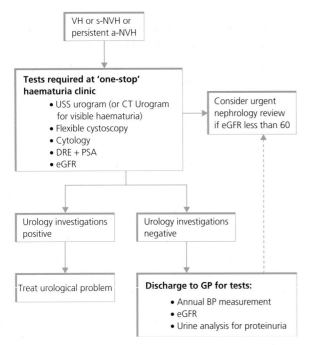

Figure 2.1 OSH investigations.

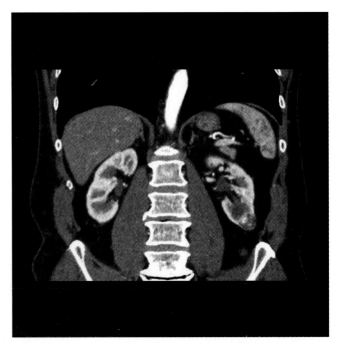

Figure 2.2 Renal tumour on CT scan.

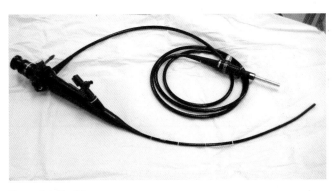

Figure 2.3 Flexible cytoscope.

the scope (see Figure 2.3). The patient is brought to hospital as a day-patient, and after informed consent has been obtained, is placed in the supine position on a couch. Antiseptic is applied to the glans penis or female urethral meatus, followed by injection of lignocaine gel into the urethra. The flexible cystoscope is then introduced, and the urethra, prostate (in men), bladder neck and bladder are inspected. Before the procedure, a urine dipstick should be checked to exclude UTI. Flexible cystoscopy is good at diagnosing bladder lesions such as transitional cell carcinoma (TCC), which have a characteristic, fronded appearance. It can also diagnose cystitis, bladder calculi, and urethral strictures and obstruction caused by the prostate.

Ultrasound of the urinary tract

Ultrasound scanning (USS) is a cheap, minimally invasive, sensitive investigation for investigating the upper tracts of the haematuria patient. It should be performed for all patients with visible haematuria, as well as those with symptomatic non-visible haematuria

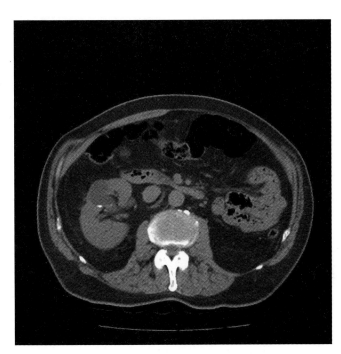

Figure 2.4 A complex cyst in the right kidney seen on CT.

and asymptomatic, persistent non-visible haematuria. Cystic and solid masses can be distinguished, as well as acoustic shadows cast by calculi. Obstruction of the kidneys can also be seen in the form of hydronephrosis. Ultrasound is often performed in conjunction with a plain x-ray of the abdomen, as ultrasound can sometimes miss calculi and approximately 90% of urinary tract stones are radio-opaque.

Low-risk, younger patients who have asymptomatic, self-limiting, non-visible haematuria may not necessarily need to be investigated with cystoscopy although cystoscopy is still recommended – this should be decided on a case-by-case basis. This is only the case if the patient is less than 40 years old, and if they are considered to be in the low-risk category for bladder cancer. Risk factors include smoking and pelvic radiotherapy. If no cystoscopy is performed, the urine should be sent for cytology.

Further management of haematuria

If a urological cause for the haematuria is found, further treatment will then be planned. Where the cystoscopy reveals a bladder tumour then urgent admission for transurethral resection of the bladder tumour (TURBT) is required. The further management of bladder tumours is discussed in Chapter 9 on bladder cancer. A renal tumour detected on ultrasound should be further staged by urgent CT urogram (see Figure 2.4) and then the options for management decided following urgent discussion at the local multidisciplinary tumour group meeting (MDT) (and see Chapter 10 on renal cancer).

If no urological cause is found, the patient should be kept in the primary-care setting and should have annual blood pressure, eGFR and urine analysis for proteinuria by the GP. If the eGFR is abnormal or proteinuria is discovered, urgent referral to a nephrologist should be considered.

The management of patients presenting with haematuria as an emergency

Sometimes, patients with visible haematuria may present as an emergency. The most extreme example of this is those patients who have clot-retention.

If a patient presents with a history of prior macroscopic haematuria with painful retention of urine and a palpable bladder, they should be referred to the urology department for evaluation urgently. Once arrived in hospital, their urgent management should be urethral catheterisation with an irrigating ('three-way') catheter, at least 20F in size. This allows both the relief of the retention, as well as the possibility to irrigate the bladder, with the intention of stopping the bleeding. Irrigating catheters allow better evacuation of blood clots than the standard two-way catheters. The patient should be admitted to the ward, and undergo bladder irrigation until the urine clears. Ultrasound of the renal tract should be performed and in most cases a rigid cystoscopy under general anaesthesia will be required if there is continued bleeding because a poor view is usually obtained with a flexible cystoscope under these circumstances. Cystoscopy and bladder washout will also be required where the bleeding is persistent and this may include diathermy of any bleeding points. The patient should give consent for transurethral resection of any tumour which might be found during this procedure.

Further reading

Anderson J, Fawcett D, Feehally J, Goldberg L, Kelly J and MacTier R. BAUS/RA Guidelines July 2008. *Joint Consensus Statement on the Initial Investigation of Haematuria*. www.bauslibrary.co.uk/PDFS/BAUS/haematuria_consensus_guidelines_July_2008.pdf.

Khadra MH, Pickard RS, Charlton M, Powell PH and Neal DE. A prospective analysis of 1,930 patients with hematuria to evaluate current diagnostic practice. *J Urol* 2000 Feb; 163(2): 524–7.

Oosterlinck, van der Meijden, Sylvester, Böhle, Rintala, Narvón, Lobel. *Guidelines on TaT1 (Non-Muscle Invasive) Bladder Cancer*. European Association of Urology Guidelines 2006. http://www.uroweb.org/nc/professional-resources/guidelines/online/.

Stenzl, Cowan, De Santis, Jakse, Kuczyk, Merseburger, Ribal, Sherif, Witjes. *Guidelines on Metastatic and Muscle-invasive Bladder Cancer*. European Association of Urology Guidelines 2009. http://www.uroweb.org/nc/professional-resources/guidelines/online/.

CHAPTER 3

Bladder Outflow Obstruction

James Allan

OVERVIEW

- Differentiating between storage and voiding symptoms is an important part of patient assessment
- Investigations for lower urinary tract symptoms (LUTS), including symptom scores and flow rates, can help decide the best treatment options
- Conservative management of benign prostatic hyperplasia (BPH) with medical therapy is now the mainstay of treatment
- Surgical management of BPH will include transurethral resection of prostate (TURP) and laser resection/ablation
- Other causes of LUTS include strictures, and detrusor dysfunction

Bladder outflow obstruction (BOO) due to benign prostatic enlargement (BPE) is an extremely common clinical presentation. Thirty per cent of men in their fifties and 50% of men in their eighties have moderate to severe lower urinary tract symptoms (LUTS). Ten per cent of men aged 60 and 25% of men at 80 have a diagnosis of benign prostatic hyperplasia suggesting the reluctance of men to consult their GP regarding symptoms (Figure 3.1).

The interwoven nomenclature used in bladder outflow obstruction may be confusing and the relationship between the various terms is demonstrated in Figure 3.2 which also includes definitions.

Symptoms

Lower urinary tract symptoms (LUTS) are divided into storage and voiding symptoms. The term voiding is used rather than obstructive to reflect the fact that poor detrusor function rather than bladder outflow obstruction may be the cause of such symptoms. Voiding symptoms include decreased flow, hesitancy, intermittency, a significant post-void residual, a post-void dribble, prolonged voiding, and abdominal straining. Storage symptoms include urinary frequency, nocturia, urgency and urge incontinence; the term storage is used rather than irritative as this would imply an inflammatory process (Table 3.1).

The differential diagnosis of LUTS caused by BPH is important and reflects the need for accurate assessment in the primary care setting. Possible alternative diagnoses are bladder and prostate cancer, urinary tract infections, overactive bladder syndrome (OAB), urethral strictures and neurological disease affecting the lower urinary tract.

Assessment

The assessment of a patient includes a focused history and examination, a validated symptom score (such as the International Prostate Symptom Score, IPSS), urine analysis and prostate specific antigen (PSA) when appropriate. The history should assess general health as general medical conditions such as diabetes, cardiovascular disease and fluid intake may cloud the diagnostic picture. Clinical examination must involve a focused examination of the external

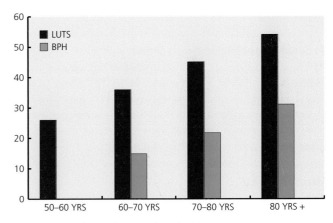

Figure 3.1 Prevalence of LUTS and BPH in UK men.

Table 3.1 Lower urinary tract symptoms.

Voiding symptoms	Storage symptoms
Weak urinary stream	Frequency
Prolonged voiding	Nocturia
Abdominal straining	Urgency
Hesitancy	Urge incontinence
Intermittency	
Incomplete bladder emptying	
Terminal and post-void dribbling	

ABC of Urology, Third Edition.
Edited by Chris Dawson and Janine M. Nethercliffe.
© 2012 John Wiley & Sons, Ltd. Published 2012 by John Wiley & Sons, Ltd.

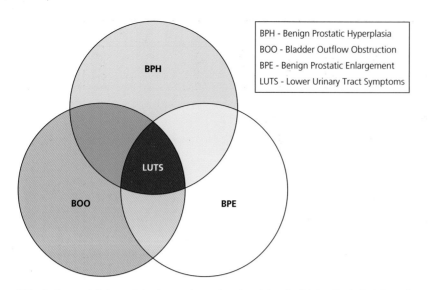

BPH - Benign Prostatic Hyperplasia
BOO - Bladder Outflow Obstruction
BPE - Benign Prostatic Enlargement
LUTS - Lower Urinary Tract Symptoms

BPH = Benign prostatic hyperplasia - increase in number of prostate cells. This is a histological diagnosis.

BPE = Enlargement of the prostate gland, which may be due to benign prostatic hyperplasia.

BOO = Obstruction of the bladder outflow, regardless of cause. BPO (benign prostatic obstruction) is BOO secondary to BPE.

Figure 3.2 Urinary tract terminologies.

genitalia and a digital rectal examination (DRE). DRE enables the examiner to make a rough estimate of prostate size and more importantly will probably detect locally invasive prostate cancer. Urinalysis is performed to ascertain the presence of haematuria, infection or diabetes. Historically symptom scores, such as the IPSS, were regarded as tools of clinical trials but they now form an essential part of the primary assessment. Validated symptom scores are useful to assess the severity of symptoms and response to treatment (Figure 3.3).

Prostate specific antigen (PSA)

PSA is prostate specific not disease specific. There are two reasons for measuring PSA in a patient with LUTS: to manage prostate cancer risk, and to identify patients with BPH whose disease is more likely to progress. Age adjusted PSA values are used to manage prostate cancer risk (Table 3.2). In benign disease progression is more likely in patients with a PSA of greater than 1.5 ng/ml.

Urodynamics

The simplest test is a flow rate study and an ultrasound scan of the bladder after voiding to assess bladder emptying. A normal maximum flow rate is considered to be about 25 ml per second and a significantly reduced flow is less than 10 ml per second. Ideally a patient empties their bladder after voiding but commonly a small residual is left.

Table 3.2 PSA age specific values.

Age	Normal PSA range
40–49	<2.5
50–59	<3.5
60–69	<4.5
70–79	<6.5

In order to assess complex symptoms and bladder dysfunction more invasive urodynamic investigation may be required. The detrusor pressure can be assessed by measuring intravesical pressure and rectal pressure, using water filled lines and pressure transducers. The detrusor pressure is then calculated by subtracting the rectal (intra-abdominal) pressure from the intravesical pressure. Thus in the patient with LUTS physicians can diagnose and distinguish high-pressure low-flow obstructed systems, detrusor dysfunction or the atonic bladder. Urodynamics are also used to demonstrate the ability of the bladder to provide stable storage of urine or conversely bladder instability and storage symptoms. This is important in patient selection for surgery and predicting surgical outcomes.

Treatment of bladder outflow tract obstruction

After evaluation patients should be offered treatment based on the severity of their symptoms, the bother they cause, and the general health of the patient.

Indications for urological referral and intervention include acute urinary retention, bladder stones and large post-void residuals leading to obstructive nephropathy or recurrent infections and severe symptoms failing medical management (Box 3.1).

Box 3.1 **Indications for urological referal and intervention**

Acute urinary retention
Obstructive nephropathy
Large post-void residual volume causing UTIs
Bladder stones
Failure of medical treatment

	Not at all	Less than 1 time in 5	Less than half the time	About half the time	More than half the time	Almost always	Your score
1. Incomplete emptying Over the past month, how often have you had a sensation of not emptying your bladder completely after you finish urinating?	0	1	2	3	4	5	
2. Frequency Over the past month, how often have you had to urinate again less than 2 hours after you finished urinating?	0	1	2	3	4	5	
3. Intermittency Over the past month, how often have you found you stopped and started again several times when you urinated?	0	1	2	3	4	5	
4. Urgency Over the past month, how difficult have you found it to postpone urination?	0	1	2	3	4	5	
5. Weak stream Over the past month, how often have you had a weak urinary stream?	0	1	2	3	4	5	
6. Straining Over the past month, how often have you had to push or strain to begin urination?	0	1	2	3	4	5	

	None	1 time	2 times	3 times	4 times	5 times or more	Your score
7. Nocturia Over the past month, how many times did you most typically get up to urinate from the time you went to bed unitl the time you got up in the morning?	0	1	2	3	4	5	

| **Total IPSS score** | | | | | | | |

0–7 = mildly symptomatic; 8–19 = moderately symptomatic; 20–35 = severely symptomatic

Figure 3.3 International prostate symptom score.

There are four treatment options: conservative management, medical management, surgery or a catheter (Box 3.2).

Box 3.2 **Treatment options for bladder outflow obstruction**

Watchful waiting
Alpha-blockers
5-Alpha-reductase inhibitors (5ARIs)
Combination therapy
Phytotherapy
Surgery
Catheter

Conservative management

For the patient with mild symptoms reassurance and a trial of conservative measures may be satisfactory. Possible conservative measures are advice on fluid intake, reduction of caffeine and alcohol, bladder retraining and continence products.

Medical management of bladder outflow obstruction

In recent years dramatic advances in the medical treatment available to patients with bladder outflow obstruction has greatly improved non-surgical management. Drug treatment is the initial treatment for most patients with alpha blockers and 5-alpha-reductase inhibitors being the main drugs of choice. Relatively recently it was proposed that obstruction in men with symptomatic BPH comprised both static and dynamic elements. The static element of obstruction is the mechanical obstruction caused by the enlarged prostatic adenoma and the dynamic element is the tone of the prostatic smooth muscle. Thus two different pharmacological routes for symptom relief have evolved namely relaxing the prostate or shrinking the prostate.

Alpha-blockers

These work by relaxing the muscle tone in the bladder neck and prostate. All alpha-blockers have similar efficacy but the older, less uro-selective drugs tend to have greater side effects. They have a rapid onset of action and tend to improve symptoms in 70 % of men. However, with time, symptoms progress and there is no evidence that they lower the risk of long-term symptom progression or acute events. The side effects of alpha-blockers are shown in Box 3.3.

Box 3.3 **Side effects of alpha-blockers**

Postural hypotension 10%
Lethargy 10%
Gastrointestinal disturbance 8%
Nasal congestion 8%
Ejaculatory dysfunction 12%

5-Alpha-reductase inhibitors (5ARIs)

5ARIs reduce the size of the prostate over months by inhibiting the conversion of testosterone into its active metabolite dihydrotestosterone. They are recommended for prostates greater than 30 cc in size. Approximately 20% of men experience significant symptomatic improvement. They also lower the risk of symptom progression, acute retention and the need for surgical intervention by 50%. Their side effect profile is extremely low with approximately 5% of men experiencing erectile dysfunction and 5% with decreased libido. As they reduce the glandular volume by approximately 50% it must be remembered that they reduce PSA by 50% as well.

Combination therapy

Combination therapy with an alpha-blocker and a 5ARI is recommended for men with severe symptoms and risk factors for progression. There have been two long-term clinical trials of combination therapy. These have suggested a slightly greater reduction in symptom scores for those patients on combination therapy rather than monotherapy with an alpha-blocker or a 5ARI. Combination therapy also reduces the risk of acute retention and surgical intervention. Over four years it was shown that 10% of men on monotherapy had symptom progression compared to 5% of men on combination therapy.

Phytotherapy

Saw Palmetto, extracted from the berries of the American dwarf palm, is the most popular and widely available herbal medication used to treat symptomatic BPH. Other agents tried are extracts from African plum tree, pumpkin seeds, rye pollen, South African star grass, stinging nettles, and pine flower. There is a general paucity of good quality data to champion the use of phytotherapy.

Anticholinergic drugs

These have a significant role to play in patients with significant storage symptoms and overactive bladder. Caution should be used in patients with high post-void residuals or severe voiding symptoms. Storage symptoms commonly cause greater bother to patients than voiding symptoms and need treating to improve quality of life.

Surgical management of bladder outflow obstruction

Transurethral resection of the prostate (TURP)

When medical treatment fails or symptoms demand it patients may be offered surgery. Transurethral resection of the prostate remains the gold standard treatment for most patients with lower urinary tract symptoms and is the benchmark that all other treatments are measured against. Ninety per cent of men experience good symptomatic relief after a TURP.

TURP involves surgically removing the periurethral and transitional zones of the prostate to relieve obstruction. This is performed by electrocautery through endoscopic instruments introduced via the urethra. Tissue is resected in small chips until the obstruction is removed and a satisfactory channel is established. Patients are catheterised for approximately 2–3 days and may be an in-patient for this period. A full recovery takes between 4 and 6 weeks. There is a small (less than 1%) risk of postoperative mortality. The possible complications of TURP are seen in Box 3.4.

Box 3.4 **Complications of TURP**

Medical complications 5%
Urinary tract infections 2%
Blood transfusion 6%
Retrograde ejaculation 70%
TUR Syndrome 2%
Impotence 8%
Incontinence 1%
Failure to void 5%

Laser surgery

In recent years laser surgery has increased in popularity and a number of techniques have been described.

Holmium laser enucleation of the prostate (HoLEP)

Holmium laser enucleation of the prostate removes the prostate from its capsule in several large pieces. These pieces are then removed endoscopically from the bladder. The potential advantages are that a catheter is only required overnight, a shorter hospital stay, greater resection weights compared to TURP and less bleeding. HoLEP is now achieving results that are comparable to TURP.

Laser ablation of the prostate

The laser vaporises prostatic tissue creating a channel through the prostate. Several types of laser including holmium, thulium and green light, have been used to achieve ablation or vaporisation. At present the long-term results of laser ablation do not seem to parallel those of the gold standard TURP or HoLEP.

There have been numerous alternative therapies such as balloon dilatation, urethral stents, microwave therapy and needle ablation that have not stood the test of time and are presently not recommended.

Management of acute urinary retention (AUR)

Acute retention is managed with catheterisation. Most men with simple acute retention are offered a trial without catheter after being prescribed an alpha-blocker for at least two days. Those patients failing a trial without catheter should be considered for surgical intervention. Men with AUR with complications such as hydronephrosis, chronic retention, obstructive nephropathy and bladder stones should be considered for surgical intervention

Other causes of bladder outflow obstruction

Urethral strictures

Strictures may cause outflow tract obstruction. The aetiology of strictures may be infective, traumatic, iatrogenic or idiopathic. The signature flow rate shows a plateau with a prolonged voiding cycle. Treatment of a short stricture is by endoscopic urethrotomy. Longer, complex or recurrent strictures may be difficult surgical problems and may require complex reconstruction.

Bladder neck dysfunction

Bladder neck dysfunction is sometimes seen in younger men. It is common to see a high bladder neck that fails to relax during voiding. The prostate is normal on DRE. Treatment may either be pharmacological with an alpha-blocker or surgical with a bladder neck incision. Bladder neck incision may create retrograde ejaculation so men wishing to remain fertile often prefer alpha-blocker treatment rather than undergo this procedure.

Further reading

Roehrborn CG, Siami P, Barkin J et al. The effects of combination therapy with dutasteride and tamsulosin on clinical outcomes in men with symptomatic benign prostatic hyperplasia: 4-year results from the CombAT study. *Eur Urol* 2010 Jan: 57; 123–31.

Madersbacher S, Marszalek M, Lackner J, Berger P, Schatzl G. The long-term outcome of medical therapy for BPH. *Eur Urol* 2007 Jun; 51(6): 1522–33.

NICE. Management of lower urinary tract symptoms in men. Clinical guideline 97. May 2010. www.nice.org.uk/nicemedia/live/12984/48557/48557.pdf.

McConnell, JD, Roehrborn, CG, Bautista OM et al. The long-term effect of doxazosin, finasteride, and combination therapy on the clinical progression of benign prostatic hyperplasia. *NEJM* 2003; 349: 2387–98.

CHAPTER 4

Urinary Incontinence

Janine M. Nethercliffe

OVERVIEW

- Urinary incontinence is a distressing symptom which can have a significant impact on a person's quality of life
- Patients may present with a mixture of symptoms and a thorough history and examination are required to determine the nature of the underlying problem
- Urodynamic assessment is the mainstay of diagnosis of detrusor overactivity
- Stress incontinence is the commonest type of incontinence in women and results from weakness of the urinary sphincter
- Women should only be considered for surgery for stress incontinence where conservative measures have failed to result in sufficient improvement

Definition

The bladder's function is to store urine at low pressure and to empty to completion at a socially acceptable time. The bladder is a muscular sac that fills with urine and the muscle relaxes as the bladder fills to keep the pressure low. The urine is held in by the urinary sphincter, which is a circular muscle around the outlet of the bladder. In order for voiding to occur, the sphincter has to relax and the detrusor muscle contract so that the pressure within the bladder is greater than the sphincter muscle. This is normally a coordinated process controlled by centres in the brain stem. (see Figure 4.1).

Urinary incontinence, defined by the International Society of Continence as 'the involuntary leakage of urine that is a social or hygienic problem', is a distressing symptom, which can have a significant impact on a person's quality of life.

Classification of urinary incontinence

Main types of incontinence

- Urge
- Stress
- Continuous
- Overflow

ABC of Urology, Third Edition.
Edited by Chris Dawson and Janine M. Nethercliffe.
© 2012 John Wiley & Sons, Ltd. Published 2012 by John Wiley & Sons, Ltd.

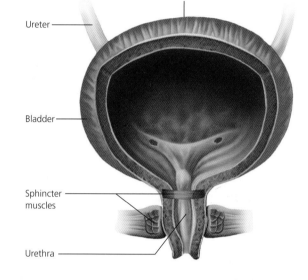

Figure 4.1 Anatomy of the bladder.

Urinary incontinence can be described either by the symptom or by the underlying mechanism. There is much overlap in these two classifications.

Urge incontinence (symptom) is leakage accompanied by or immediately preceded by urgency. The underlying mechanism is normally increasing detrusor pressure, detrusor overactivity (mechanism).

Stress incontinence (symptom and mechanism) is leakage on effort or exertion. The underlying mechanism is normally a weakened sphincter.

Mixed incontinence (symptom) in which both urge and stress symptoms are experienced.

Nocturnal Enuresis (symptom) is leakage of urine during sleep. Common in children and may be a symptom of an overactive detrusor muscle.

Post-micturition dribbling (symptom) is leakage experienced immediately following urination often due to pooling of urine in urethra.

Continuous incontinence (symptom) is the continuous leakage of urine.

Overflow incontinence (mechanism) is the leakage of urine due to obstruction and a full bladder.

Functional incontinence (mechanism) is where the bladder works normally but because of impaired mobility or mental functioning the person urinates inappropriately.

Urge incontinence and stress incontinence are the most common forms and this chapter will concentrate on their causes and management.

Diagnosis and investigation of urinary incontinence

History and examination

History

- Mobility
- Nature and duration of symptoms
- Other illnesses
- Cultural and social factors
- Lifestyle factors, such as fluid intake
- Previous surgery
- Mental status
- Medication
- Sexual function
- Bowels
- Treatment expectations
- Patient's fitness for surgery if applicable

'The bladder is an unreliable witness', and patients may present with a mixture of symptoms which obscure the clinical picture and make it difficult to determine the predominant type of incontinence.

For these reasons it is important to take a thorough history which should include previous surgery and any neurological conditions (remembering that incontinence may be the first presenting symptom for a neurological condition such as multiple sclerosis). Nocturnal enuresis or continuous incontinence is often apparent from the history. Drinking habits, family history and medication must all be included. A bladder diary is a useful tool in the initial assessment of the patient and can help clarify symptoms and assess drinking habits.

Examination must be thorough, not only concentrating on the lower urinary system but also looking for systemic illness. Examination may reveal a full bladder, which might lead to the diagnosis of overflow incontinence. Where appropriate, assessment of the pelvic floor should be carried out by an experienced doctor, with results clearly recorded. Vaginal prolapse, pelvic floor assessment and the presence of stress incontinence during coughing or straining should be looked for. The perineal skin condition should also be assessed. It is an intimate examination that should not be repeated unnecessarily especially by inexperienced junior doctors. The woman's consent for a pelvic examination must always be obtained. Rectal examination to assess the prostate in men should be included and rectal examination also allows anal tone to be assessed when neuropathy is suspected.

Examination

- General wellbeing and fitness for treatment
- Mobility
- Abdominal examination
- Pelvic examination
- Rectal examination

Investigations

Urinalysis should be performed on all new patients. Further evaluation depends on whether any doubt remains over the diagnosis and the likely treatment. There is no point in conducting an invasive investigation on an elderly man if he is too unfit for any other treatment than a long-term catheter.

Flow rates and post-micturition scans are an easy investigation that can be carried out in the out-patient setting. Pad testing and bladder diaries can be performed or directed easily by a nurse prior to the consultation.

Urodynamic assessment, although the term includes flow rates, is a term normally applied to pressure flow tests. These involve fine catheters inserted into the bladder and the rectum. Pressure transducers allow the pressures to be measured within the bladder and the abdomen. Subtraction of the abdominal pressure from the vesical pressure gives the detrusor pressure. This investigation is the mainstay of diagnosis of detrusor overactivity. It can be combined with imaging, and filling the bladder with contrast allows imaging of the bladder during filling, and the bladder, bladder neck and urethra during voiding. Urodynamic assessment also allows the bladder to be imaged during straining and coughing to assess bladder neck descent for assessment of stress incontinence. With appropriate transducers urethral pressures can also be measured although this is usually a research tool rather than standard clinical practice. It is to be remembered that the test must try to replicate the patient's symptoms as much as possible, understanding that is a very artificial situation; this can be overcome by ambulatory urodynamics, which has a better pick-up rate for detrusor overactivity. (see Figure 4.2).

Cystoscopy is performed if there are symptoms (such as haematuria or pain) to suggest intravesical pathology, or if a fistula is suspected.

Investigations

- Urinalysis
- Frequency/volume chart
- Flow rate and bladder scan
- Pad testing
- Urodynamics
- Endoscopy
- Other imaging

Urge incontinence

Urge incontinence is the most common type of incontinence in men and the elderly population. The patient experiences an intense

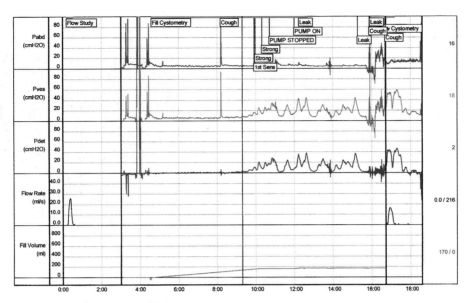

Figure 4.2 Urodynamics tracing showing detrusor overactivity.

and sudden need to pass urine, which can occur spontaneously or be triggered by a change in position, running water, and other situations.

Urge incontinence is caused by the detrusor muscle contracting inappropriately. This leads to an intravesical pressure that exceeds that of the sphincter causing leakage to occur. If the pressure does not exceed that of the sphincter the person will still experience urgency but will not leak (see Figure 4.3).

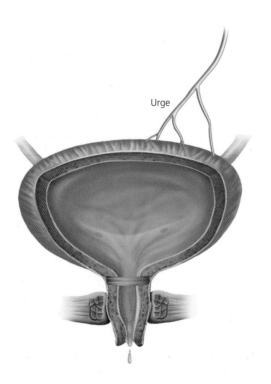

Urge

Figure 4.3 Urge incontinence is the leakage of urine due to detrusor contraction.

Overactive bladder is the term used for the condition with or without incontinence and is estimated to affect about 50 million people in Europe. It is normally termed neuropathic when the cause is due to neurological conditions such as spinal injury, and non neuropathic where either the cause has not been identified, or is related to local causes within the bladder.

Causes of urge incontinence

- Cystitis
- Bladder stone
- Obstruction of the bladder, such as an enlarged prostate
- Idiopathic detrusor overactivity, also known as non-neuropathic detrusor overactivity
- Neuropathic detrusor overactivity, e.g. spinal injury, multiple sclerosis, Parkinson disease, spina bifida and stroke

Specific investigations and management of urge incontinence

Cystometry is the diagnostic tool that allows assessment of the inappropriate detrusor contractions. However, first line treatments are often given without the necessity of this invasive test.

Treatment of urge incontinence

- Resolve underlying pathology
- Lifestyle changes
- Anticholinergics
- BOTOX
- Sacral nerve stimulation
- Surgery

Treatment of this condition should always include resolving any causative pathology present, e.g. urinary tract infection or a bladder stone. Conservative measures such as: good fluid intake of non-caffeinated drinks; the planning and timing of voiding; and avoiding letting the bladder get over-filled can decrease the incontinence episodes.

The next line of management is normally anticholinergic medication. This group of drugs blocks receptors on the detrusor muscle which respond to acetylcholine from the muscarinic nerves to the bladder, and which are responsible for bladder contraction.

Botulinum toxin works in a similar way to anticholinergic drugs but, rather than block the receptors on the bladder, it prevents the release of acetylcholine in the nerve endings, resulting in a more powerful effect. The results of this treatment are very promising but there is a significant risk (25%) that the patient will need to self-catheterise following the treatment. The treatment is performed via a flexible cystoscope with local anaesthetic gel: 200–300 units of toxin are injected, in 1 ml volumes (10 units per ml) into the wall of the bladder via a specially designed needle which allows the correct depth of penetration. Often a blister is seen under the urothelium during injection. The procedure is normally well tolerated. The effect of the toxin lasts about 6–9 months, so the treatment has to be repeated.

Sacral nerve stimulation is a recognised treatment for refractory urge incontinence. It is based on modulating the S2-4 sacral nerves, the main nerves responsible for bladder contraction.

Surgery is often the last resort for patients who have intractable urge incontinence. A clam cystoplasty involves dividing the bladder open 'like a clam' and placing a piece of intestine into the opening. This manoeuvre increases the capacity of the bladder and possibly divides the 'abnormal nerves'. The intestinal piece is a low-pressure segment that can act like a diverticulum during a contraction to prevent leakage. The operation is not without its complications, including stone formation, infection, metabolic upset, and possible long-term risk of malignant change. Patients having this procedure will require annual surveillance cystoscopy. Urinary diversion is also a surgical option in certain cases.

Stress incontinence

Stress incontinence is the commonest type of incontinence in women. It is caused by weakness of the urinary sphincter causing leakage when extra pressure is placed on the bladder e.g. by coughing or sneezing. In women it normally reflects pelvic floor weakness and/or sphincter damage associated with childbirth, age, menopause, previous hysterectomy, or obesity (see Figure 4.4).

Causes of stress incontinence

- Age
- Previous childbirth
- Hysterectomy
- Obesity
- Trauma
- Previous prostate surgery

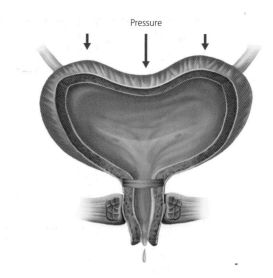

Figure 4.4 Stress incontinence is leakage of urine from increase pressure outside the bladder.

Specific investigations and management of stress incontinence

Treatment of stress incontinence in women

- Pelvic floor exercises
- Weight loss
- Stop smoking
- Avoid constipation
- Surgery

The National Institute for Health and Clinical Excellence (NICE) has published guidelines for the treatment of women with stress incontinence. It strongly recommends conservative measures in the first instance. Physiotherapy with pelvic floor exercises for at least three months can improve the strength of the pelvic floor and sphincter as well as teaching certain techniques that can decrease the leakage. Other conservative measures include weight loss, stopping smoking and avoiding constipation. Women should only be considered for surgery where conservative measures have failed to result in sufficient improvement.

Colposuspension and autologous pubovaginal slings are tried and tested operations. A number of minimally invasive procedures have come and gone due to poor long-term results, but in the last decade the situation has changed with the advent of tension-free mid-urethral tapes. This is now the most common operation for stress incontinence in women, the principal being the placement of a synthetic tape behind the posterior wall of the urethra to form a hammock. There are a number of different tapes and approaches available (see Figure 4.5).

Another minimally invasive procedure performed for stress incontinence is the injection of bladder neck bulking agents, where a synthetic material is injected into the wall of the urethra to augment the sphincter. The long-term results for this procedure are not as good as for the sling procedures.

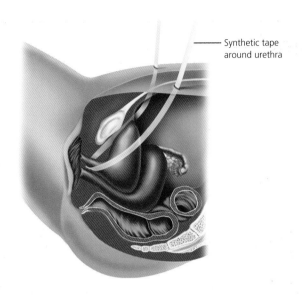

Synthetic tape
around urethra

Figure 4.5 Tension-free vaginal tape. Figures shows position of synthetic tape around urethra.

Artificial urinary sphincters placed around the bladder neck can be used in women. In extreme cases of incontinence following earlier failed procedures, urinary diversion may be the only other option; especially in cases where there may be significant disability such as with advanced multiple sclerosis.

Stress incontinence in men

Stress incontinence is less common in men and is commonly found with a history of surgery or trauma. Investigations should include video-urodynamics and endoscopy to assess sphincter coaptation.

Treatment of stress incontinence in men is based on increasing the resistance of the outflow. The sphincter can be augmented by injection of a bulking agent. This procedure has been found to have a variable effect and is not regarded as a permanent solution. The insertion of an artificial sphincter does have good results in men. It is inserted around the bulbar urethra and has a reservoir and a pump mechanism that inflates a cuff around the urethra increasing the resistance and preventing leakage.

Mixed incontinence

This is not normally seen in men but is common in women who often present with both stress leakage and urgency. Sometimes the urgency is due to detrusor overactivity and sometimes it is habitual or results from urine leaking into the urethra. Urodynamics is the key investigation to determine the true cause of the urgency as it is important to exclude detrusor overactivity in these patients as stress incontinence surgery can worsen these symptoms.

Continuous incontinence

Sometimes known as total incontinence, continuous incontinence occurs when the bladder cannot store urine at all and results in continuous leakage. This normally results from a defect in the bladder from birth or from trauma, either from surgery or childbirth causing a fistula. In developed countries with good obstetric care the commonest cause of vesico-vaginal fistula is from gynaecological surgery.

Overflow incontinence

This is caused when the bladder becomes obstructed. The bladder fills up and when it is very full, pressure in the bladder increases and periodically exceeds that of the sphincter, leading to leakage. It is more common in men who are more likely to have an obstructed bladder due to an enlarged prostate gland.

Causes of bladder obstruction

- Enlarged prostate
- Previous surgery, for example incontinence surgery
- Bladder stones
- Urethral stricture
- Constipation

Further reading

2nd International Consultation on Incontinence. *Recommendations of the International Scientific Committee: Evaluation and Treatment of Urinary Incontinence, Pelvic Organ Prolapse and Faecal Incontinence.* P. Abrams, K.E. Andersson, W. Artibani, L. Brubaker *et al.* July 2001: 1079–114.

National Institute for Health and Clinical Excellence. *Urinary Incontinence: The management of urinary incontinence in women.* 2006, London: NICE.

2006 EAU Guidelines on Urinary Incontinence, J Thuroff, P Abrams, KE Anderson, W Artibani, E Chartier-Kastler, C Hampel, Ph Van Kerrebroeck.

CHAPTER 5

Urological Emergencies

William J.G. Finch

OVERVIEW

This chapter outlines how to recognise and deal with common urological emergencies seen in hospital and the community:

- Acute urinary retention
- Renal colic
- Testicular torsion
- Paraphimosis
- Priapism

Urological emergencies are seen commonly by doctors in training, emergency physicians and general practitioners. Although life-threatening urological emergencies are rare they are an important part of a doctor's knowledge base. Acute urinary retention, renal colic, testicular torsion, paraphimosis and priapism will be discussed in this chapter. We hope to arm the reader with the information needed to recognise and deal with these urological emergencies.

Retention of urine

Urinary retention is one of the commonest urological emergencies, mainly affecting elderly men. Urinary retention is the inability to urinate and therefore empty the bladder. It may be acute or chronic and either spontaneous or precipitated by another problem e.g. urinary tract infection (UTI) or constipation.

The exact cause of acute urinary retention is unclear, however several different conditions may contribute to it and these can be broadly divided into four major categories (see Box 5.1). Obstruction may be due to mechanical or dynamic causes. Inflammation, swelling and oedema are often a result of urinary tract infection. Several neurological conditions can lead to retention, and over-distension of the bladder reduces the ability of the bladder to contract normally.

Treatment of acute retention requires urgent catheterisation (Box 5.2) which should bring immediate relief of the

---

Box 5.1 Categories of acute urinary retention

Obstructive

- Mechanical obstruction
  - Benign prostatic hyperplasia
  - Urethral stricture
  - Constipation
  - Pelvic mass
- Dynamic obstruction
  - Increase in smooth muscle tone due to postoperative pain and drugs

Inflammatory

- Urinary tract infection
- Prostatitis

Neurological

- Interruption of sensory or motor innervation to the bladder
  - Spinal cord injury
  - Multiple sclerosis
  - Pelvic surgery

Over-distension

- Post-anaesthesia
- High alcohol intake
- Drugs
  - Ephedrine, pseudoephedrine
  - Antidepressants

Box 5.2 Male catheterisation top tips

- **Ensure penis is held straight** and 90° to body
- **Gently and slowly insert adequate anaesthetic gel** into urethra. Gently occlude meatus to stop gel oozing out whilst waiting
- **Talking to patient** is an excellent distraction whilst passing catheter.
- If difficulty inserting catheter – useful to **try the next size up**
- **Do not force a catheter** – always call for more experienced help
- Always **record the residual volume** of urine

ABC of Urology, Third Edition.
Edited by Chris Dawson and Janine M. Nethercliffe.
© 2012 John Wiley & Sons, Ltd. Published 2012 by John Wiley & Sons, Ltd.

patient's discomfort. It is important to record the volume of urine drained in the first 10–15 minutes; this is usually <1 litre. If urethral catheterisation in the primary care setting fails then the patient should be admitted urgently for consideration of a suprapubic catheter.

Patients with normal renal function, who have had any precipitating factors corrected, may be offered a trial without catheter usually after commencing an alpha-blocker for 2–3 days. If this trial without catheter fails, these patients are either managed with a long-term catheter, or offered prostatic surgery. The patient in many cases can be managed in primary care and referred for advice if he fails a trial without catheter.

If the volume drained is more than 1 litre this suggests chronic retention. Chronic retention is associated with less pain, may be painless, and patients often have few urinary symptoms. Classically patients describe nocturnal enuresis, which is felt to be overflow incontinence due to loss of voluntary sphincter tone during sleep.

Chronic retention may be associated with abnormal renal function and upper tract dilatation. In these cases, immediate catheterisation is essential to decompress the upper tracts and allow renal function to recover. A period of diuresis may follow requiring close monitoring of electrolytes, blood pressure and the patient's weight. A trial without catheter is not appropriate in these cases, and patients (if fit enough) should undergo elective prostatic surgery or else be managed with a long-term catheter. These patients should be referred urgently for admission to the urology department for monitoring and investigation.

Renal colic

Renal colic presents as severe, sudden-onset pain which the patient often describes as their 'worst pain ever'. Classically the pain starts in the flank and radiates around the front of the abdomen to the groin and sometimes to the scrotum in men and the labia in women. The pain generated by renal colic is primarily caused by the dilatation, stretching and spasm caused by acute ureteral obstruction. Nausea and vomiting is often associated with the pain and some patients will see visible blood in their urine.

Examination of the abdomen is often unremarkable with only a few patients demonstrating tenderness at the loin or groin. Commonly patients are unable to find a comfortable position with the pain and appear restless. This is in sharp contrast to the patients with a peritonitic abdomen who try to lie absolutely still.

Urinalysis will reveal non-visible blood in over 85% of renal colic cases. If no blood is demonstrated, other diagnoses such as appendicitis, diverticulitis, salpingitis and ruptured abdominal aortic aneurysm need serious consideration.

Routine blood tests should be sent to include renal function, and pregnancy must be excluded in women of childbearing age.

Imaging for renal colic has moved away from plain x-ray and intravenous urogram (IVU) in recent years. Non-contrast CT scans of the abdomen and pelvis are quick to perform and report and are now readily available in most hospitals (Figure 5.1). They have been shown to be more accurate than IVU in detecting stones and may provide an alternative diagnosis with a comparable radiation dose.

Initial treatment of a patient with renal colic involves resuscitation with fluid, anti-emetics and analgesia. Non-steroidal anti-inflammatory drugs such as diclofenac should be used before opiate-based analgesia as they provide more effective pain relief with fewer side effects.

The chance of a patient passing the stone is related to its size and position within the ureter (Table 5.1).

The detailed management of stones is considered in chapter 12.

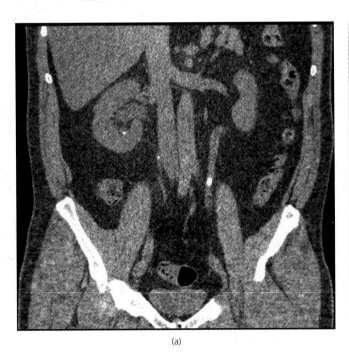
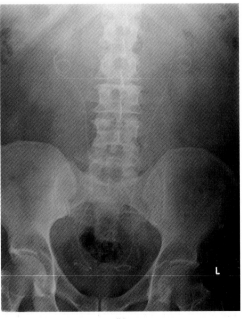

(a) (b)

Figure 5.1 (a) Unenhanced CT scan showing bilateral ureteric stones; (b) bilateral ureteric stones with ureteric stents.

Table 5.1 Spontaneous stone passage rates for stone size.

Stone size	Chance of stone passing spontaneously
<4 mm	90%
4-6 mm	50%
>6 mm	20%

An infected and obstructed kidney is a true urological emergency. Typically these patients are unwell, with a history of rigors and pyrexia, and can deteriorate rapidly. Once diagnosed they need urgent percutaneous decompression with nephrostomy, vigorous resuscitation with intravenous antibiotics and fluids, and intensive clinical monitoring. These patients should be referred to hospital as an emergency.

Testicular torsion

Testicular torsion is a urological emergency. Prompt diagnosis and surgical exploration within 4–6 hours of the onset of pain is critical to preserve the testis.

Testicular torsion results from a twisting of the spermatic cord, which impedes blood flow to the testis and impairs venous drainage, resulting in oedema, ischaemia and necrosis. There is a bimodal age distribution with the first peak at age 1–2 years and the second much higher peak in teenage years. Torsion is relatively uncommon in adults over 40.

The most common reason for this is a malformed tunica vaginalis, which normally attaches the upper pole of the testis to the posterior scrotum, fixing it in place. When the tunica vaginalis instead extends over the whole testis, fixing it in a horizontal position, this is called a 'bell-clapper deformity', and predisposes to torsion.

The most common presentation with testicular torsion is that of pain and swelling. The history is very important in distinguishing testicular torsion from other common causes of acute scrotal pain such as epididymitis or appendiceal torsion. Testicular torsion typically has a quicker onset of pain, and patients may have had previous episodes of pain indicating intermittent torsion. Examination reveals an acutely tender swollen testicle (Figure 5.2). The testicle may be lying horizontally and sitting high in the scrotum, and some believe an absent cremasteric reflex to be diagnostic.

Urinalysis is often normal. Colour flow Doppler ultrasound may be used to demonstrate poor or absent blood flow in equivocal cases, but should not delay surgical exploration. No one sign or symptom establishes the diagnosis of torsion, but when clinical suspicion suggests testicular torsion, urgent surgical exploration of the scrotum is required.

Timing of surgical exploration of the scrotum is directly related to testicular torsion salvage rates (Figure 5.3) hence the importance of a speedy diagnosis.

Surgical treatment consists of detorting the affected testis and fixing the testis to the scrotal wall using non-absorbable sutures, or by placement within a dartos pouch. If the testis is not salvageable an orchidectomy is performed (Figure 5.4). The unaffected testicle is also explored as tunical malformations contributing to testicular torsion are often bilateral. The unaffected testis should also be fixed to the scrotal wall.

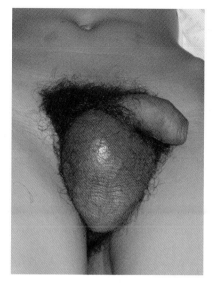

Figure 5.2 Typical presentation of acute scrotum (image with permission of Mr O Wiseman).

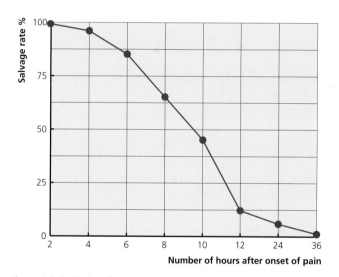

Figure 5.3 Testicular salvage rates depend on time to presentation.

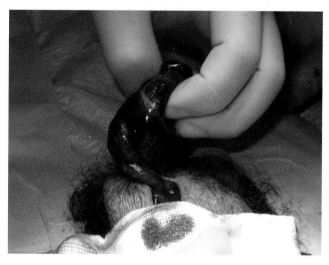

Figure 5.4 Testicular torsion (image with permission of Mr O Wiseman).

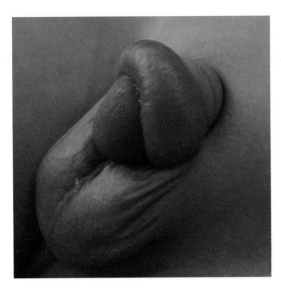

Figure 5.5 Paraphimosis.

Paraphimosis

Paraphimosis is a common condition that occurs in uncircumcised men. It occurs when the foreskin becomes fixed in the retracted position and cannot be reduced therefore constricting venous return from the glans penis and resulting in swelling of the glans (Figure 5.5).

Paraphimosis is often related to a prior phimosis, with a constriction band of the prepuce acting as a tourniquet, preventing retraction as well as venous and lymphatic drainage. The most common cause however is iatrogenic, with medical staff failing to replace the foreskin following urethral catheterisation.

Without early intervention paraphimosis can result in ulceration, and necrotic changes in the preputial skin and glans penis.

Various treatments are used in a sequential manner after adequate analgesia, which may involve a penile nerve block. Manual decompression involves compressing the glans to reduce the oedema and then attempting to replace the foreskin over the glans penis.

A dorsal slit performed by a urologist may be required if other techniques fail. This divides the preputial constriction band and allows reduction of the foreskin. Formal circumcision is the definitive treatment and will prevent any further episodes. This is usually performed at a later date because the prepuce may be swollen and ulcerated, making for a difficult circumcision procedure.

Priapism

Priapism is defined as penile erection persisting beyond, or unrelated to, sexual stimulation. There are two types of priapism. Low-flow priapism or ischaemic priapism results from decreased venous and lymphatic drainage of the corpus cavernosae. High-flow or non-ischaemic priapism results from unregulated arterial blood flow often related to trauma. The main complication of priapism is

Table 5.2 Common causes of priapism.

Idiopathic	
Haematological	Sickle-cell disease
	Leukaemia
	Thrombophilia
Neurological	Spinal cord lesions
Medications for erectile dysfunction	Intracaverosal papaverine
	Intracavernosal prostaglandin E1
	Intraurethral alprostadil
Other drugs	Antihypertensives
	Antipsychotics
	Antidepressants
	Alcohol and cocaine

erectile dysfunction and the aim of prompt management is to avoid this and potential psychological morbidity.

Low-flow priapism is painful, is more common, and most cases are as a result of medication or drug use (Table 5.2); the incidence is significantly higher in men with sickle cell disease or blood dyscrasias. The decreased venous and lymphatic drainage can lead to thrombosis and further ischaemia, resulting in fibrosis of the corpora cavernosae and erectile dysfunction.

High-flow priapism is less common, and often less painful. It often follows perineal or penile trauma (commonly straddle type injuries), producing a cavernosal artery laceration, subsequent arteriovenous fistula, and thus unregulated arterial blood flow within the corpora cavernosae of the penis.

Treatment of priapism depends on differentiation between low-flow and high-flow types. The definitive distinction can be made by penile blood gas analysis, aspirated from the corpus cavernosum, whilst simultaneously assessing and treating underlying causes (e.g. sickle cell disease).

Primary treatment for low-flow priapism involves aspiration and irrigation of the corpora and possibly intracavernosal injection of phenylehprine, which requires cardiac monitoring. If these conservative measures are unsuccessful, a surgical shunt between the corpora cavernosa and spongiosa is required and potentially immediate penile prosthesis insertion. Treatment for high-flow priapism is less urgent and cases can be observed prior to arteriography and selective embolisation with good functional outcomes.

Further reading

Emberton M and Fitzpatrick JM. The Reten-World survey of the management of acute urinary retention: preliminary results. *BJU Int* 2008; 101s3: 27–32.

Masarani M and Dinneen M. Ureteric colic: new trends in diagnosis and treatment. *Postgrad Med J* 2007; 83: 469–72.

Kapoor S. Testicular torsion: a race against time. *Int J Clin Pract* 2008; 62: 821–7.

Broderick GA, Kadioglu A et al. Priapism: pathogenesis, epidemiology and management. *J Sex Med* 2010; 7: 476–500.

Little B and White M. Treatment options for paraphimosis. *Int J Clin Pract* 2005; 59: 591–3.

CHAPTER 6

Subfertility and Male Sexual Dysfunction

Helen Hegarty

OVERVIEW

- Refer the subfertile couple early to a specialist centre if risk factors have been identified
- Assisted reproduction techniques achieve a conception rate of about 20% per cycle
- Identify and treat risk factors for erectile dysfunction (ED) and don't forget psychogenic ED as a cause
- It is reasonable to try a phosphodiesterase inhibitor (such as sildenafil) in straightforward ED
- There are a variety if treatments for ED and ejaculation dysfunction and the patient should be counselled by a specialist to discuss these options

Infertility is defined as the failure to conceive after regular unprotected intercourse for two years in the absence of reproductive pathology.

Subfertility

Eighty-four per cent of couples will successfully conceive within the first year of trying; this decreases with increasing maternal age. The main causes of reduced fertility are outlined in Table 6.1.

Assessment of the infertile couple

A detailed history should be taken from both patients, concentrating on history, especially history of STDs and past surgical procedures, age, smoking and alcohol intake.

Reversible risk factors should be corrected where possible and couples with no history of other risk factors should be encouraged to continue trying for a further 12 months before any further treatment is offered. If risk factors, such as known hormonal, endocrine or genetic abnormalities or undescended testes, are identified, further investigation should be offered early. Further investigation is undertaken usually at a specialist centre and involves semen analysis, male hormone screen (which includes testosterone,

follicle stimulating hormone (FSH), luteinising hormone (LH) and prolactin), ovulation assessment, sexually transmitted disease (STD) swabs, assessment for fallopian tubal damage, and uterine and cervical mucus tests.

Normal parameters for semen analysis are taken from the World Health Organization reference values (Table 6.2) and should be repeated if abnormal.

Assessment of the female patient is more complex. A hormone screen (which includes progesterone, LH, FSH and prolactin) and a transvaginal scan can diagnose a variety of endocrine and hormonal pathologies and demonstrate the number of developing follicles. It will also pick up abnormalities of the ovaries and uterus, such as fibroids. Hysterosalpingography (HSG) can diagnose tubal occlusion.

Treatment of male factor infertility

Table 6.3 summarises the treatment for male factor infertility. If anti-sperm antibodies are identified, treatment with corticosteroids may help but usually assisted conception techniques are required. Varicoceles are often diagnosed in the presence of male subfertility; however there is no evidence that surgical correction increases conception rates for the subfertile man. This is also true for the

Table 6.1 The causes of male and female factor infertility.

Causes of male factor infertility	Causes of female factor infertility
Idiopathic	Failure of ovulation (includes hormonal imbalances resulting from disease of the ovary, hypothalamus and pituitary)
Undescended testis	Pelvic inflammatory disease
Functional sperm disorders	Scarred/obstructed fallopian tubes
Ejaculation disorders	Endometriosis
Testicular injury	Idiopathic
Obstructive azoospermia	Drugs (chemotherapy, marijuana, smoking, alcohol), toxins
Drugs (chemotherapy, marijuana, smoking, alcohol), toxins	Endocrine and genetic and congenital disorders
Systemic disease (diabetes, renal failure, cystic fibrosis)	Uterine (fibroids, polyps, adenomyosis)
Hormone, endocrine and genetic disorders	Hostile cervical mucus
	Maternal age >35

ABC of Urology, Third Edition.
Edited by Chris Dawson and Janine M. Nethercliffe.
© 2012 John Wiley & Sons, Ltd. Published 2012 by John Wiley & Sons, Ltd.

Table 6.2 WHO reference values for seminal analysis.

Standard tests	Normal values
Volume	2 ml or more
pH	7.2–7.8
Sperm concentration	20×10^6 spermatozoa/ml
Total sperm count	40×10^6 spermatozoa or more
Morphology	30% or more with normal morphology
Motility	50% or more with forward progression or 25% or more with rapid progression within 60 mins after collection
Vitality	75% or more live
White blood cells	Fewer than 1×10^6/ ml

Table 6.3 Treatment of male factor infertility.

Cause	Treatment
Oligospermia	Correct hormone imbalance
	Cease toxic drugs
	Empirical treatment with clomiphene
	Assisted conception
Azoospermia	Obstructive – surgical correction
	Non-obstructive – correct hypogonadotrophism, exclude pituitary tumour, identify toxins
	Assisted conception
Testosterone deficiency	Do not give ectopic testosterone, consider gonadotrophic drugs
Hypogonadotrophic hypogonadism	Gonadotrophic drugs
Ejaculatory dysfunction	Try adrenergic drugs if no previous bladder outflow surgery
	Electroejaculation/vibroejaculation

undescended testis, although orchidopexy may be indicated to facilitate earlier detection of malignant change in the undescended testis.

Treatment of female factor infertility

Table 6.4 shows the treatment of female factor infertility. Women who take anti-oestrogens such as clomifene need to be counselled about the increased risk of multiple pregnancies.

Assisted reproduction involves sperm extraction directly from the testis or epididymis or vas deferens. Assisted conception involves in-vitro fertilisation (IVF), which is associated with pregnancy rates of about 20%. Other forms of treatment involve depositing sperm directly into the uterus (interauterine insemination, IUI) and

Table 6.4 Treatment of female factor infertility.

Cause	Treatment
Hypothalamic pituitary dysfunction (ex polycystic ovaries)	Anti-oestrogens (clomifene or tamoxifen)
	Metformin
	Laparoscopic ovarian drilling
	Gonadotrophins
Hypoprolactinaemia	Dopamine agonist (bromocriptine)
Tubal occlusion	Surgery
Uterine fibroids or adhesions	Surgery
Endometriosis	Laparoscopic ablation and adhesiolysis
Idiopathic	Assisted conception

injecting a single spermatozoon directly into the oocyte (intracytoplasmic sperm injection, ICSI). In some cases, donor insemination needs to be considered.

Counselling should also be included in the treatment plan as couples can find this process very stressful. In addition, all decisions about treatment need to involve both partners with a detailed explanation of the success rates and complications so that an informed decision can be made.

Male sexual dysfunction

Erectile dysfunction (ED) can be defined as the persistent inability to achieve or maintain an erection sufficient for penetration and sexual intercourse. Penile erection depends on an intact nervous system and adequate and correctly responding vasculature as well as the ability to become aroused. Parasympathetic nerves originating from S2–4 are important for erection and sympathetic nerves from T11–L2 serve ejaculation. One in ten men have ED and the incidence increases with age.

Audiovisual stimuli act in the brain to activate the nervous pathways described above and cause an erection. The cavernosal nerve is stimulated and this activates the erectile tissue of the corpora cavernosa to fill with blood by relaxation of the cavernosal smooth muscle and opening of the vascular space. This compresses the tissue against the tunica albuginea and occludes venous outflow, thus maintaining the erection (Figure 6.1). Ejaculation is achieved by tactile stimulation of the glans (via the pudendal nerve) and stimulation of the sympathetic nerves causing contraction of the smooth muscle of the epididymis, vas deferens and the secretory glands of the prostate, which emits sperm and seminal fluid into the prostatic urethra. The bladder neck simultaneously closes, the external sphincter opens and the bulbocavernosus muscle contracts rhythmically to allow emission of the semen. Nitric oxide (NO) and prostaglandin E1 (PGE1) cause a decreased availability of intracellular cavernosal calcium levels and thus are important in cavernosal smooth muscle relaxation and thus forming a rigid erection (Figure 6.2).

The causes of erectile dysfunction are listed in Table 6.5. Evaluation of the patient with ED centres on identifying the potential cause and treating this where possible. Important factors in the

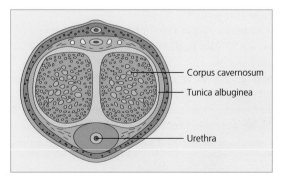

Figure 6.1 Transection of the penis demonstrating the erectile tissue (corpora cavernosa) and the stiff tunica albuginea, which occludes the outflow of blood and helps maintain the erection.

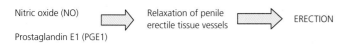

Figure 6.2 Transmitters causing erection.

Table 6.5 Causes of erectile dysfunction.

Idiopathic	
Psychological	Depression, anxiety, stress
Age	
Vascular pathology	Hypertension, smoking, hypercholesterolaemia
	Failure of the veno-occlusive mechanism (venous leak)
Peyronie's Disease	
Neurogenic	Spinal cord disorders, pelvic radiotherapy, multiple sclerosis, Parkinson's disease
Drugs/toxins	Anti-hypertensives, anti-depressants, anti-androgens, anti-convulsants alcohol, statins
Endocrine disorders	Diabetes, hypogonadism, pituitary tumour
Previous surgery and trauma	Radical prostatectomy, pelvic fracture
Systemic disease	Renal failure, cirrhosis

history include age, duration of onset, history of pelvic surgery or trauma and radiotherapy, history of hypertension, hyperlipidaemia, diabetes and medications. It is important to note that erectile dysfunction is a presenting complaint in other serious underlying illnesses and investigation is important to rule out conditions such as hypertension, subclinical cardiovascular disease and diabetes. Smoking and alcohol consumption are important. The presence of morning erections is a good indicator that the physiology is intact and the cause is likely to be non-organic.

Examination focuses on excluding Peyronie's disease by the palpation of penile shaft plaques, a neurological examination and prostate assessment. The location and size of the testes is important and the bulbocavernosus reflex can be checked by squeezing the glans and looking for anal sphincter and bulbocavernosus muscle contraction (indicating an intact S2–4 pathway).

Further investigations involve:

- serum hormone screen, especially if libido is effected or if the testes are small
- nocturnal penile tumescence testing to measure nocturnal erections
- Doppler ultrasound to investigate the arterial supply
- Induction of an artificial erection to see the response to prostaglandin E1
- Cavernosography to identify venous leak.

Treatment of erectile dysfunction

In the clinic setting, if there are no specific risk factors other than age and arteriopathy or diabetes, the clinician may try a phosphodiesterase inhibitor (such as sildenifil) to see if the patient responds. If not he may then be referred on to an andrologist. Before instigating assessment and treatment for ED, the patient needs to be deemed fit enough to engage in sexual intercourse.

Psychogenic ED requires the help of a psychosexual counsellor, and the patient may attend for this with or without his partner. Adjuvant treatment with oral medication or PGE1 medication may also be used.

Medical therapy for ED

Oral medication involves phosphodiesterase type-5 inhibitors (PDEI5), such as sildenafil and vardenafil, which act by enhancing the smooth muscle relaxation and thus erection. The dosage can be titrated upwards until a response is seen and there are also longer-acting medications available such as tadalafil. The patient should be counselled about potential side effects such as headache, flushing and visual disturbance and those patients taking nitrates must avoid these medications.

Testosterone replacement should be considered in those with low testosterone. Testosterone replacement leads to suppressed spermatogenesis. Its effects need to be carefully monitored and the prostate specific antigen (PSA) should be checked beforehand as testosterone is contraindicated in prostate cancer.

Medications used on/in the penis

Synthetic PGE1 (alprostadil) can be administered directly into the corpora cavernosa or trans-urethrally to cause an erection directly. It does not rely on arousal (as is the case for the oral medications). Priapism is a risk and the patient needs to be warned about this and advised to seek treatment if the erection is prolonged and unwanted. Injectable alprostadil may be associated with fibrosis of the tunica albuginea over time.

Vacuum devices

These use a constriction band at the base of the penis and a vacuum device which traps blood in the erectile tissue. It can be cumbersome to some patients and may cause bruising.

Penile prostheses

Insertion of either malleable or inflatable penile devices (Figure 6.3) involve destroying the erectile tissue but do provide a dependable erection where other treatments have failed or are not suited to the patient and his partner. Once inserted, the patient cannot go back to using the other treatment methods and this needs to be made clear. The surgery should be performed by surgical andrologists who perform a large number of these procedures to minimise the complications, which include infection, erosion, extrusion and auto-inflation.

Treatment of ejaculation disorders

These can include premature ejaculation, retrograde ejaculation and anejaculation. In those who do not ejaculate, occlusion of the vas deferens needs to be excluded and surgically corrected. In premature ejaculation topical local anaesthesia to the glans can help, as can PDE5 inhibitors. Other treatments include condoms containing a local anaesthetic, squeezing of the glans penis to retard ejaculation, and the use of antidepressant medications (selective

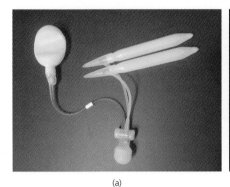

(a)

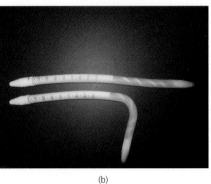

(b)

Figure 6.3 a/b Inflatable and malleable penile prostheses.

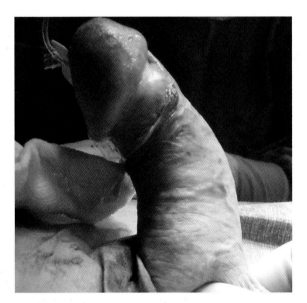

Figure 6.4 Patient with Peyronie's disease undergoing artificial erection during Nesbit procedure. Note the typical dorsal curvature of the penile shaft.

serotonin reuptake inhibitors). Retrograde ejaculation is usually the result of alpha-blockers, such as tamsulosin, being used to treat bladder outflow obstruction (BOO). In this case the drug may simply be stopped. It is also a common consequence of surgery for BOO and in this case nothing can be done. The patient can be reassured that it is not detrimental to his health. In other cases oral adrenergic drugs may be tried.

Treatment of Peyronie's disease

Peyronie's disease is caused by the formation of fibrous tissue plaques on the tunica albuginea causing a deviation in the erect penis and pain (Figure 6.4). If pain is a factor, no definitive treatment should be attempted until at least 6–12 months after the pain has ceased. If intercourse is difficult or not possible the patient may be treated initially with a trial of vitamin E (200 mg TDS), tamoxifen or POTABA during the acute phase. Once the deformity has stabilised for at least six months, and if penetrative intercourse is not possible, a Nesbit procedure may be performed where the penis is straightened by removing small segments of the tunica albuginea from the opposite side of the plaque. Other procedures include plaque incision and grafting.

Further reading

CG11: Fertility. National Institute for Health and Clinical Excellence (NICE). 25 Feb 2006, updated 30 Mar 2010.
Cooper TG, Noonan E and von Eckardstein S. World Health Organization Reference Values for Human Semen; 2009.
WHO manual, 3rd edition, 1992.

CHAPTER 7

The Management of Adult Urinary Tract Infection

Richard Cetti and Suzie Venn

OVERVIEW

- UTIs are a common and significant burden on the health economy
- The sensitivity of a combined nitrite and white cell dipstick for diagnosing UTI is approximately 88%
- Asymptomatic bacteriuria in a catheterised patient does not require treatment
- Pregnant women with asymptomatic bacteriuria should be treated to prevent pyelonephritis and risk of miscarriage
- UTI in a man raises the possibility of an underlying functional or anatomical abnormality
- Men with UTIs and women with recurrent UTIs, or patients with persistent non-visible haematuria/sterile pyuria, should be referred for urological investigation.
- An infected obstructed kidney is a urological emergency and requires prompt resuscitation and drainage

Definition

Not just the presence of, but also the inflammatory response to, a micro-organism infection of the urine that can involve the upper or lower urinary tract.

The strict criteria of $>10^5$ bacteria/ml on MSU is no longer required for diagnosis. Current recommendations for the diagnosis of UTI on MSU have been published by the EAU and are summarised in Table 7.1.

Incidence

In the absence of good European data, the US have estimated that UTIs are responsible for over 7 million consultations annually, and approximately 15% of all community antibiotic prescriptions. Importantly they also account for at least 40% of all hospital-acquired infections, with increasing problems of antibiotic resistance.

ABC of Urology, Third Edition.
Edited by Chris Dawson and Janine M. Nethercliffe.
© 2012 John Wiley & Sons, Ltd. Published 2012 by John Wiley & Sons, Ltd.

Table 7.1 Recommended criteria for the diagnosis of UTI on urine culture.

Type of UTI	Urine culture
Acute uncomplicated UTI	$>10^3$ cfu/ml
Acute uncomplicated pyelonephritis	$>10^4$ cfu/ml in women
Complicated UTI	$>10^5$ cfu/ml in women
	$>10^4$ men
Recurrent UTI	$<10^3$ cfu

cfu = colony forming units

Aetiology

Several factors predispose to developing a UTI, those related to the host, and those to an infecting organism. These are summarised in Figure 7.1.

Most UTIs are caused by faecal-derived bacteria, the most common being Gram-negative bacilli such as *Escherichia coli*, and species of the genera *Klebsiella* and *Proteus*. *E. coli* is the causative pathogen in approximately 70–95% of cases of uncomplicated UTI. As with many Gram-negative bacteria they have pili on their cell surface, which aid attachment to the urothelium. This helps prevent them being washed out with urine flow, and contributes to their ability to ascend and cause upper tract infections (Figure 7.2). The loss of this mechanical flushing effect of the antegrade flow of urine in urinary tract obstruction can result in urinary stasis and promote bacterial proliferation. Other host factors that protect against UTI include the presence of vaginal commensal bacteria. Lactobacilli metabolise glycogen to lactic acid creating an inhospitable environment for uropathogens. Atrophy of vaginal tissue following the menopause results in a loss of lactobacilli. This is the rationale behind the use of topical oestrogens and live yogurt as treatment for recurrent UTI. Any foreign body is a focus for infection; this includes indwelling catheters and stents (Figure 7.3). The majority of patients with long-term catheters will develop bacteriuria. It is important to remember, however, that only those with a symptomatic infection should be treated with antibiotics to prevent the development of bacterial resistance.

Classification

Urinary tract infection can be classified depending upon the involvement of the upper or lower urinary tract and whether it

WHAT ARE THE CAUSES?

Breach of bladder lining

Foreign body

Calculi

Diabetes mellitus

Immunocompromise

Urinary tract obstruction

Female-pregnancy/post-menopausal

HOST vs ORGANISM

Virulence factors

Figure 7.1 Factors that contribute to UTI.

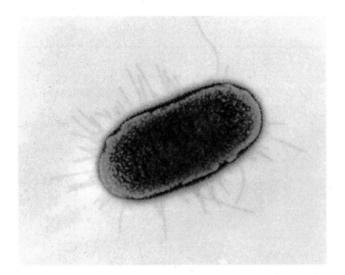

Figure 7.2 Transmission electron micrograph of *Escherichia coli* negatively stained to enhance contrast. Note the projecting pili. Courtesy of Wadsworth Center, New York State Department of Health.

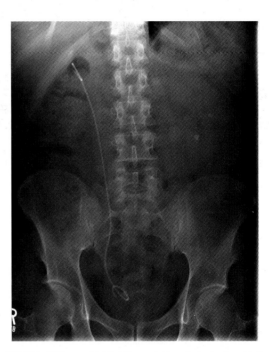

Figure 7.3 Plain KUB x-ray highlighting a right ureteric stent and left renal calculi.

is complicated or uncomplicated. The features of upper and lower tract involvement are outlined in Table 7.2.

An uncomplicated UTI is one occurring in a patient with a structurally and functionally normal urinary tract. A complicated UTI conversely is one occurring in the presence of an underlying anatomical or functional abnormality. The distinction between the two is important because it has implications with regard to acute management and further follow-up. There are several factors that can aid suspicion and direct further investigation (Box 7.1).

Management of uncomplicated UTI in women

Almost half of all women will experience one UTI during their lifetime. Diagnosis is made on history and urine investigations. Routine urine analysis by dipstick is an easy bedside test. It utilises

a reagent strip with various impregnated marker pads with enzyme dependent colour changes, specific to among others: blood, protein, white blood cells and nitrites (Figure 7.4). Nitrites do not occur normally in the urine, but many species of Gram-negative bacteria can convert urinary nitrates to nitrites. The sensitivity of a combined

Table 7.2 Features of upper and lower urinary tract infection.

Lower urinary tract	Upper urinary tract
Frequency	Fever
Dysuria	Loin pain
Suprapubic pain	Vomiting
Haematuria	

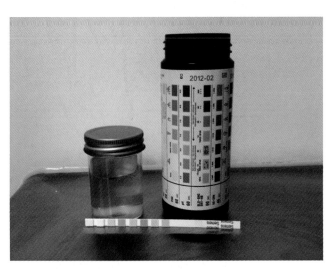

Figure 7.4 Urine dipstick.

nitrite and white cell dipstick for diagnosing UTI is as high as 88%. Urine microscopy and culture are not routinely required for women with uncomplicated UTI. It should be undertaken if there are risk factors for a complicated urinary tract infection, the woman has recurrent episodes, or has not responded to antibiotic treatment, depending on local guidelines. Recent studies have shown rising patterns of resistance, in particular to trimethoprim and co-amoxiclav. The patient should have routine primary care follow-up to ensure that the treatment has been successful. No further investigation is required unless the patient develops signs of upper tract infection, a complicated UTI, recurrent infections or is pregnant (Box 7.2).

Occasionally patients may present with symptoms of a UTI, but have no growth of organisms on microscopy and culture, despite having persistent white cells on urinalysis – sterile pyuria. Sensitivity of microscopy for Gram-stained bacteria is approximately 90%, but is dependent on patients' fluid intake, collection technique and transport times. In the presence of persistent symptoms, non-visible haematuria or sterile pyuria, the patient should be referred for urological assessment to rule out underlying malignancy or atypical infection such as TB.

Pyelonephritis and the management of sepsis

Pyelonephritis defines an upper tract infection of the kidney and renal pelvis. It is a clinical diagnosis based on the presence of loin pain and pyrexia, invariably with a leucocytosis, positive urinalysis and signs of sepsis. The patient may well describe a preceding lower urinary tract infection. Differential diagnoses include: appendicitis, cholecystitis, pneumonia and generalised septicaemia from a distant source. Those patients who have fever, but who are not systemically unwell, can be managed in primary care. EAU guidelines recommend an oral quinolone antibiotic for 7 days as first-line therapy.

If a patient, however, shows signs of sepsis (Box 7.3) and is systemically unwell they should be admitted for intravenous antibiotics and further investigation with a plain KUB (kidneys, ureters and bladder) x-ray and ultrasound of the renal tract to rule out an upper tract obstruction, calculus disease or, rarely, gas around the kidney suggestive of an emphysematous pyelonephritis.

Recurrent UTI

This is defined as more than two infections in 6 months, or three within 12 months. These patients are managed in the acute episode as for an uncomplicated UTI, but must be further investigated to rule out a cause of bacterial persistence, for example, urinary tract calculi, poor bladder emptying or a neoplastic process in the bladder. Patients should have plain KUB x-ray imaging and an ultrasound scan of the urinary tract, including post-void residual. A flexible cystoscopy should be considered in patients over 40 years of age or those with persistent non-visible haematuria.

When reversible causes have been ruled out these patients can be managed in several ways. They should firstly be advised on lifestyle changes as outlined in Box 7.4. Low dose prophylactic antibiotics (LDPA) may reduce recurrences by up to 95% compared with placebo. The optimal schedule or duration of LDPA is not known, but should involve the rotation of antibiotics to prevent bacterial resistance.

Special circumstances

UTI in pregnancy

The rates of bacteriuria are similar in pregnant and non-pregnant women. However, a number of physiological and anatomical changes occur during pregnancy, which put a woman at increased risk of developing a UTI from this. The bladder is displaced anteriorly and superiorly by the enlarging uterus, which may result in poor urinary flow and bladder emptying. In addition there is dilatation of the upper tracts caused by a combination of mechanical obstruction and smooth muscle relaxation due to progesterone. Approximately 4% of pregnant women have asymptomatic bacteriuria, of whom 20–40% will develop pyelonephritis during their pregnancy with the attendant risks to mother and baby. Women are therefore screened throughout pregnancy, with bacteriuria treated promptly with antibiotics.

UTI in men and prostatitis

UTI is less common in men due to the length of the male urethra, and therefore its diagnosis should raise the possibility of underlying complications, such as bladder outflow obstruction (Figure 7.5). Urological evaluation is required. In addition to the routine investigations outlined for women, a man should have a detailed history taken of lower urinary tract symptoms, a digital rectal examination of the prostate and assessment of flow rate and post-void residual. When assessing the prostate particular attention should be made to the size, texture, symmetry and presence of tenderness suggestive of prostatitis.

Prostatitis is infection or inflammation of the prostate and can therefore occur both in the presence of UTI and also with sterile urine. A useful investigation to determine a bacterial prostatitis is by performing a modified Stamey test, and sample different parts of the urinary stream before, during and after prostatic massage. A confirmed bacterial prostatitis should be treated with a 6-week course of a quinolone antibiotic. Inflammatory prostatitis is a spectrum of the chronic pelvic pain syndrome and should be managed appropriately.

Epididymo-orchitis

Epididymitis causes pain and swelling of the epididymis. It is usually acute in onset and unilateral. In young men the usual cause is sexually transmitted and *Chlamydia trachomatis* is isolated in approximately two thirds of these cases. Orchitis in isolation is less

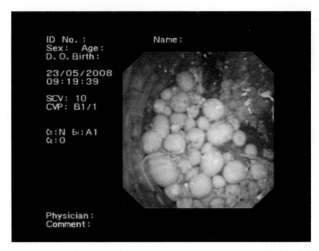

Figure 7.5 Multiple bladder calculi in a man with UTIs and prostatic bladder outflow obstruction.

common. The most common type is mumps orchitis which develops in 20–30% of post-pubertal patients undergoing mumps infection. When the inflammatory process affects both the epididymis and the testis the term epididymo-orchitis is used. Treatment with a quinolone antibiotic should be first line unless *Chlamydia* has been detected in which case treatment should be with doxycyline.

Infection in the presence of an obstructed upper tract

This is a urological emergency, usually associated with calculus obstruction of the ureter. The obstructed side must be drained expeditiously after initial resuscitation of the patient and administration of intravenous antibiotics. In the septic patient this is best achieved with a percutaneous nephrostomy sited under local anaesthetic, using radiological guidance. This mitigates the need for a general anaesthetic required for retrograde stenting, ensures a direct measure of urine output and drainage from the affected kidney, and provides pus for microbiology analysis. The cause of the obstruction can be dealt with at a later date when the patient is well.

Further reading

Naber KG, Bishop MC, Bjerklund-Johansen TE et al (2007). *Guidelines on the Management of Urinary and Male Genital Infections.* European Association of Urology, http://ww.eau.org.

Foxman B. Epidemiology of urinary tract infections: incidence, morbidity, and economic costs. *Am J Med* 2002 Jul 8; 113 Suppl 1A: 5S–13S.

Devillé WL, Yzermans JC, van Duijn NP et al. The urine dipstick test useful to rule out infections. A meta-analysis of the accuracy. *BMC Urol* 2004 Jun 2; 4: 4.

Williams GJ, Macaskill P, Chan SF et al. Absolute and relative accuracy of rapid urine tests for urinary tract infection in children: a meta-analysis. *Lancet Infect Dis* 2010 Apr; 10(4): 240–50.

Albert X, Huertas I, Pereiró II et al. Antibiotics for preventing recurrent urinary tract infection in non-pregnant women. *Cochhrane Database Syst Rev.* 2004; (3): CD001209.

CHAPTER 8

Prostate Cancer

Simon R.J. Bott and Stephen E.M. Langley

OVERVIEW

- Prostate cancer is the most common solid malignancy in men
- Established risk factors for prostate cancer are increasing age, ethnicity, and heredity
- Prostate cancer is usually asymptomatic at presentation and detected because of raised PSA
- Most national and international urological organisations do not currently recommend population based PSA screening
- Radical prostatectomy, external beam radiotherapy, and brachytherapy are all equally effective treatments for men with localised prostate cancer

---

Introduction

Prostate cancer is the most common solid malignancy in men and is diagnosed in 36 000 men per annum in the UK. While for some it is an indolent disease, it remains the second leading cause of male cancer deaths, after lung cancer.

There are three established risk factors for prostate cancer: increasing age, ethnicity and heredity. One in ten cases is truly hereditary. If one first-degree relative is diagnosed the risk is at least doubled. If two or more first-degree relatives are affected, the risk increases 5- to 11-fold.

Presentation

Prostate cancer is usually asymptomatic at presentation and is diagnosed by prostate specific antigen (PSA) screening. Urinary symptoms (hesitancy, poor flow, incomplete emptying) secondary to bladder outflow obstruction are usually due to benign prostate hyperplasia, unless there is extensive cancer within the prostate. Less than a fifth of men present with symptoms of metastatic disease, including bone pain, spinal cord compression, malaise, weight loss and anaemia.

A PSA blood test should only be performed after a patient has been made aware of the advantages and disadvantages of the test

---

ABC of Urology, Third Edition.
Edited by Chris Dawson and Janine M. Nethercliffe.

and the possible treatment options (see Figure 8.1). A digital rectal examination is performed in all men concerned about prostate cancer, as most cancers are found in the peripheral zone of the prostate, adjacent to the rectum, and tumours >0.2 ml may be palpable. An abnormality on digital rectal examination (DRE) or an elevated age-specific PSA are indications for prostate biopsies.

Transrectal ultrasound (TRUS) guided prostate biopsies are undertaken using local anaesthesia and following antibiotic prophylaxis. A TRUS probe is placed per rectum and 8–12 biopsies are directed at the areas most likely to contain prostate cancer. Areas that feel or appear abnormal on TRUS are also sampled. Most prostate cancers are not visible on ultrasound, consequently TRUS biopsies miss 10–20% of prostate cancers. Men with a suspicion of prostate cancer, in whom TRUS biopsies are negative, may be offered more extensive and systematic sampling using a template biopsy technique (Figure 8.2). In men who have had previous negative or equivocal TRUS biopsies, in whom a suspicion of prostate cancer remains, template biopsies diagnose cancer in a further 40% of men.

PSA screening

Screening may involve: PSA testing in an asymptomatic population of men; or opportunistic PSA testing either in men requesting a test, or in men with lower urinary tract symptoms. The aim of both is to reduce prostate cancer mortality and improve quality of life.

A large ongoing European PSA screening study recently reported that after just 8 years screening the death rate from prostate cancer reduced by 20%, but was associated with a high risk of over-diagnosis and over-treatment. In this study currently 1410 men would need to be screened and 48 cases of prostate cancer would need to be treated to prevent one death from prostate cancer. Screening did result in a 41% reduction in the number of patients with metastases, so with longer follow-up the benefit of screening is likely to be greater. In a screening study from Sweden, with a median follow-up of 14 years, there was a 44% reduction of prostate cancer deaths. In this study 293 patients need to be screened and 12 treated to prevent one cancer death, a figure comparable to breast screening studies.

Currently population based PSA screening is not recommended by the World Health Organization, or most national and international urological organisations, although it remains under review.

<table>
<tr><td>

Benefits of the PSA test

- May lead to detection of cancer before symptoms develop.

- May lead to detection of cancer at an early stage when the cancer could be cured or treatment could extend life.

- Repeat PSA tests may provide valuable information aiding in a prostate cancer diagnosis.

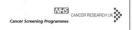
NHS CANCER RESEARCH UK
Cancer Screening Programmes

</td><td>

Limitations of the PSA test

- It is not diagnostic (a biopsy may be required).
- It is not tumour specific in the prostate.
- The PSA test result may not be elevated in some cancers and provide false reassurance.
- It may lead to the identification of prostate cancers which might not have become clinically evident in the man's lifetime.
- A single PSA test will not distinguish aggressive tumours which are at an early stage but will develop quickly from those which are not.

NHS CANCER RESEARCH UK
Cancer Screening Programmes

</td></tr>
</table>

Figure 8.1 Benefits and limitations of the PSA test (NHS Cancer Screening programmes and Cancer Research UK).

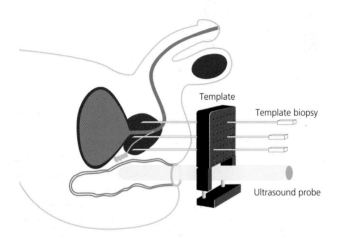

Figure 8.2 Transperineal template biopsies.

Opportunistic screening with PSA is recommended once a man has been counselled about the advantages and disadvantages of the test.

Assessment of prostate cancer

The treatment options for a man with prostate cancer depend on the PSA, grade (aggressiveness), and the stage (extent) of the disease, as well as the patient's co-morbidities.

Prostate cancer is usually a multifocal disease. Individual foci of cancer seen in prostate biopsies or TURP chippings are ascribed a grade, based on the glandular architecture from 1 to 5. The grades from the two largest foci are added to give the overall Gleason score, 2 being the least aggressive to 10 being the most aggressive. The Gleason score strongly predicts likelihood of death from prostate cancer.

The local stage of prostate cancer is assessed by the digital rectal examination, sometimes augmented by MRI scanning. In patients at risk of metastases the pelvic lymph nodes are assessed using MRI/CT and the bones by bone scintigraphy (Figure 8.3). The TNM classification is the internationally recognised staging system (Box 8.1).

In order to try and amalgamate these different parameters prostate cancer risk classifications have been developed based on PSA, Gleason grade and clinical stage that helps direct treatment (Table 8.1).

Box 8.1 TNM classification of prostate cancer (Union Internationale Contre le Cancer, 2009).

T	**Primary tumour**
T1	Clinically inapparent tumour, not palpable or visible on imaging
	T1a tumour found incidentally in ≤5% TURP chips
	T1b tumour found incidentally in >5% TURP chips
	T1c tumour identified by needle biopsy
T2	Tumour confined to the prostate
	T2a tumour involves one half of one lobe
	T2b tumour involves more than half of one lobe
	T2c tumour involves both lobes
T3	Tumour extends beyond the confines of the prostate
	T3a tumour spread beyond the prostate 'capsule'
	T3b tumour involves the seminal vesicles
T4	Tumour invades adjacent structures, including the external sphincter, rectum, levator muscles and pelvic side wall
N	**Regional lymph nodes**
N0	No nodal metastases
N1	Regional lymph node metastasis
M	**Distant metastases**
M0	No distant metastases
M1a	Non-regional lymph nodes
M1b	Bone metastasis
M1c	Other sites

Source: TNM Classification 2009.

Table 8.1 Risk stratification for men with localised prostate cancer (NICE 2008).

Risk stratification for men with localised prostate cancer. PSA		Gleason score		Clinical stage
Low risk	< 10 ng/ml **and**	≤ 6	**and**	T1–T2a
Intermediate risk	10–20 ng/ml **or**	7	**or**	T2b–T2c
High risk	> 20 ng/ml **or**	8–10	**or**	T3–T4*

*Clinical stage T3–T4 represents locally advanced disease.

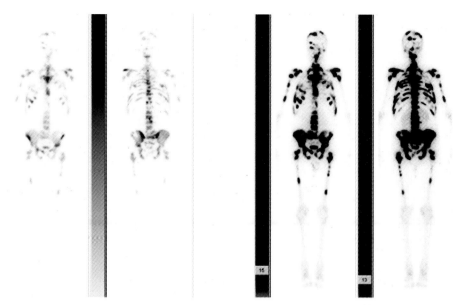

Figure 8.3 Bonescan demonstrating multiple metastases throughout the skeleton.

Management

Men diagnosed with prostate cancer may have a number of therapeutic options; all patients are therefore discussed in a multi-disciplinary meeting so the optimal treatment strategy for an individual can be offered.

Localised disease

Localised disease comprises

- men with impalpable prostate cancer and disease that is not visible with imaging (T1)
- those with disease considered confined to the prostate on rectal examination and imaging (T2)
- those confined to the prostate after pathological examination of a radical prostatectomy specimen – pT2 (Figure 8.4).

These men are potentially curable with radical therapy, including radical prostatectomy, external beam radiotherapy

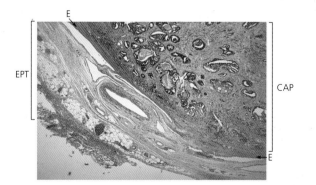

Figure 8.4 H and E stained slide showing prostate cancer (CAP) the edge or 'capsule' of the prostate (E) and the extracapsular tissue (EPT), from a radical prostatectomy specimen.

and brachytherapy. To date there is no evidence to suggest one treatment is more effective than another and all have been approved for routine clinical use by NICE. NICE also states that other treatment options, such as cryotherapy or high intensity focused ultrasound (HIFU) may be considered but only as part of a clinical trial as their long-term efficacy is uncertain.

However, prostate cancer is a slow growing tumour and therefore radical therapies normally only benefit men with a life expectancy exceeding 10 years. Furthermore, up to half of men diagnosed with prostate cancer and with a life expectancy of more than 10 years will have disease that will not affect their quality or quantity of life if left untreated and therefore the concept of active surveillance may be more appropriate.

Active surveillance

Patients with low-risk prostate cancer may be managed by active surveillance (AS), which involves close monitoring with PSA checks, and in some protocols repeat TRUS or template biopsies. This strategy aims to reduce treatment-related morbidity associated with radical therapies, whilst still allowing patients who eventually need radical therapy to receive treatment while the disease is still curable. Typically a third of these men will proceed to radical treatment either due to disease progression, or because of a change of heart by the patient. While active surveillance is suitable for many men with low-risk localised prostate cancer there is a lack of adequate predictors of higher-risk disease at the outset or markers of subsequent progression. Consequently the outcome for the patients who do subsequently receive radical treatment, in some but not all AS series, is less good than if they had received radical therapy at diagnosis.

Radical prostatectomy (RP)

Radical prostatectomy involves the surgical removal of the whole prostate and may be undertaken through an open, laparoscopic or robotic approach. The outcome from each approach is broadly speaking similar, though recovery time is faster using a minimally invasive approach.

Post-operatively the PSA should fall to unrecordable levels, but patients still require PSA monitoring for at least five years to ensure no evidence of recurrence, as for all the radical therapies. In men found to have high risk disease once the prostate has undergone pathological examination, or if the PSA starts to rise again after surgery, second-line treatment with adjuvant or salvage radiotherapy may be offered to improve cure rates.

A laparoscopic prostatectomy is a technically demanding procedure and there is a significant learning curve. The robot is reported to reduce the learning curve whilst maintaining the benefits of a shorter recovery time seen with the laparoscopic approach. Cost and availability currently restrict robotic radical to a few centres in the UK, though these are increasing year on year.

External beam radiotherapy (EBRT)

Conformal external beam radiotherapy offers men with clinically localised disease an alternative to surgery, with similar cancer outcome but with differing side effects (Table 8.2). A planning session is required prior to starting treatment; the latter is performed daily on weekdays, over a $4-7\frac{1}{2}$ week period. The radiation dose is limited by the tolerance of normal tissue in the irradiated area and UK doses are at least 74 Gray or its biologically equivalent dose.

A further modification of radiotherapy is intensity-modulated radiotherapy (IMRT). This enables improved beam shaping to anatomical contours and so reduction of the radiotherapy dose to normal structures. It therefore becomes possible to deliver a higher dose to the prostate which may reduce toxicity and improve cancer control; results from trials are awaited.

Radiotherapy treatment often includes a period of three months of androgen deprivation therapy (ADT) using a luteinising hormone releasing hormone (LHRH) agonist prior to radiotherapy. This sensitises the tumour to radiotherapy and allows the prostate to shrink (cytoreduction), enabling smaller volumes to be treated and so reducing the amount of normal tissue that is irradiated. Several large studies have confirmed the benefit of at least two years of adjuvant LHRH agonist therapy subsequent to radical radiotherapy for patients with high-grade Gleason score 8–10 tumours. This results in a significant improvement in survival over a 5-year period.

Brachytherapy

Brachytherapy involves the insertion of a radioactive source directly into the prostate, allowing a high dose of radiation to be delivered over short distance around the source, sparing normal tissue. Two types are used, iodine 125 seeds as a permanent low-dose-rate implant in the treatment of localised prostate cancer, and iridium

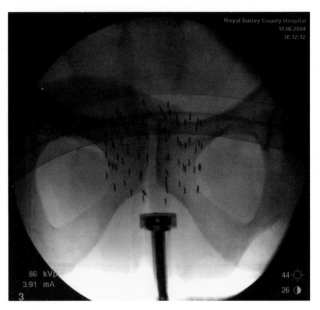

Figure 8.5 X-ray of the pelvis showing the brachytherapy seed implant in the prostate, and the TRUS probe in the rectum.

192 as a temporary, high-dose-rate implant used in conjunction with external beam radiotherapy for higher risk and locally advanced disease.

Low-dose-rate brachytherapy: iodine 125 seeds

Low-dose-rate brachytherapy is typically offered to men with low- to intermediate-risk disease and may be given alone or in conjunction with external beam radiotherapy. After an initial transrectal ultrasound scan and under general anaesthesia, 20–30 needles containing up to 120 seeds are implanted via the perineum using ultrasound guidance (Figure 8.5). This is usually performed as a day case procedure. A minimum dose of 140Gy is achieved within the prostate.

Complications of radical treatments

Whilst the cancer outcome results are similar between these three therapies there are differences in the complication rates. Complications may be related to the prostate cancer risk, patients' pre-existing symptoms and the experience of the clinical team. The reported incidence varies widely in the literature and is much debated. The main complications are shown in Table 8.2.

Other radical treatments for localised prostate cancer include high intensity focused ultrasound (HIFU) and cryotherapy.

High intensity focused ultrasound (HIFU)

HIFU uses focused ultrasound waves to heat areas in the prostate leading to coagulative necrosis. It is performed under a general anaesthetic and may also require a small transurethral resection of the prostate (TURP) to minimise post-treatment symptoms. Patients are usually discharged on the day of treatment with a urethral or suprapubic catheter for a few days.

Cryotherapy

Cryotherapy uses liquid argon to freeze the prostate. Cryoprobes are placed in the prostate under transrectal ultrasound guidance and the prostate is cooled to at least $-40°C$ leading to cell necrosis.

Table 8.2 Complications of radical treatments.

	Radical prostatectomy	External beam radiotherapy	Brachytherapy
Bowel symtoms	*	***	*
Erectile dysfunction	***	**	*
Urinary symptoms			
Frequency & urgency		***	**
Retention	*	*	***
Incontinence	***	*	*

Temperature monitors are placed at critical anatomical sites, e.g. the sphincter, to prevent damage to adjacent structures.

The procedure may be performed as a day case, and a suprapubic catheter is left in for a few days following discharge. Similarly to HIFU, patient details should be registered on a national database to comply with NICE guidance, as the clinical outcomes remain subject to review.

Locally advanced prostate cancer

Locally advanced prostate cancer includes cancer that has spread beyond the confines of the prostate, but has not metastasised. The treatment options include radical prostatectomy with extended pelvic lymphadenectomy, external beam radiotherapy with neoadjuvant and adjuvant androgen deprivation therapy (ADT) using LHRH agonists, and in some instances high-dose-rate brachytherapy.

Evidence supports improved survival in patients with locally advanced prostate cancer receiving radiotherapy with ADT versus either radiotherapy or hormone therapy alone. Radical prostatectomy case series report similar cancer outcomes to radiotherapy with ADT, though randomised trials comparing surgery with radiotherapy are currently lacking. After radical prostatectomy for locally advanced disease approximately half of men will also have radiotherapy – multimodality treatment, to improve cancer control rates.

High-dose-rate brachytherapy is less commonly used and is mainly used to treat men with high-risk localised and locally advanced disease. It is usually given after a short course of external beam radiotherapy. Hollow tubes are positioned in the prostate using ultrasound guidance with the patient under either spinal or general anaesthesia. Through these tubes the radioactive source passes delivering a dose to the surrounding tissue. The patient receives 1–3 separate doses over a 24/48 hour period, with the tubes remaining within the prostate during this time. The results using this technique are promising, though currently high-dose brachytherapy is only available in a few specialist centres.

In some patients with significant co-morbidity and locally advanced, non-metastatic prostate cancer a watch and wait policy may be adopted, with the addition of ADT at a trigger point. Evidence supports this approach in selected patients without affecting prostate cancer specific survival rates. ADT may be initiated if the baseline PSA is >50 ng/ml, or if the rate at which the PSA doubles is less than 12 months. A balance must be made between the potential side effects seen with androgen deprivation therapies and the modest, but important, reduction in unpleasant consequences of local prostate cancer progression and metastases, e.g. ureteric obstruction, spinal cord compression, painful bone metastases. As a single therapy, ADT has either no or only a small effect on survival.

Metastatic disease

The management of metastatic prostate cancer involves a multi-disciplinary approach, including urologists, oncologists, palliative care and specialist nurse support.

In 1941 Huggins and Hodges demonstrated the beneficial effect of castration and of oestrogen therapy in metastatic prostate cancer.

To this day castration, be it surgical or medical, remains the mainstay of treatment for men with metastatic disease.

Castration may be achieved surgically, either by removing the whole or just the inner part of the testes. Castration results in a rapid drop of testosterone (<12 hr) to castrate levels (<20 ng/dL). The main drawback to surgery is the psychological impact to the patient. Consequently medical castration (androgen deprivation therapy) is usually preferred, using an LHRH agonist, or more recently an LHRH antagonist.

LHRH agonists, including goserelin, leuprorelin and triptorelin, act on the pituitary gland and stop the release of LH and FSH. Testosterone levels fall to castrate levels over 2–4 weeks in 85% of individuals. Initially LHRH agonists cause a rise in LH and FSH levels 2–3 days following the first injection – this may result in a 'tumour flare' or rapid progression of tumour. The 'flare' is prevented by using a testosterone antagonist, such as cyproterone acetate or bicalutamide for approximately 3 days before and 3 weeks after the first injection. In reality in the majority of patients with low volume metastatic disease the tumour flare is only manifest by a PSA rise – the flare is potentially only an issue in men with high volume, bony metastatic disease.

LHRH analogues are administered by depot injections 1-, 3-, 6- or 12-monthly. Ongoing trials are addressing whether ADT can be administered intermittently to reduce side effects in the off-treatment periods whilst maintaining efficacy.

LHRH antagonists (abarelix and degarelix) act more quickly to lower testosterone and do not cause a tumour flare. They are used now in men with high volume metastatic disease as initial therapy, though histamine related side effects are seen and their long-term efficacy has not yet been proven.

Hormone refractory prostate cancer

After a median 24–36 months of castrate levels of testosterone the tumour develops an androgen independent state and relapses, initially seen as a rise in serum PSA. At this stage, the adrenal androgens, comprising 5–10% of total physiological serum androgen levels, may be inhibited by the addition of an antiandrogen, e.g. bicalutamide, to medical or surgical castration. Further rises in PSA may be managed by withdrawal of the antiandrogen, hydrocortisone, or oral and transdermal oestrogens.

For some men with hormone refractory prostate cancer, taxane-based chemotherapy may be offered with an improvement in quality of life as well as overall survival of about two months. Many other agents are currently under investigation as part of clinical trials. The most promising is abiraterone acetate which is currently under investigation for patients before and after chemotherapy.

Future developments

Improvements in our ability to detect and characterise significant localised disease remains critical in the management of this heterogeneous disease. More accurate risk stratification with improved imaging and biopsy techniques will reduce the number of men subjected to unnecessary treatment. For those with low- or intermediate-risk disease, targeted treatment of part of the prostate, rather than the whole gland, using focally ablative techniques may reduce the side effects seen with radical treatments. Issues regarding identification of the most important tumour to treat and how to follow up these patients still need to be addressed however.

Multi-modality treatment for more advanced tumours should improve cancer outcomes for the most high-risk patients and, as our understanding of the genetic and molecular events critical to prostate cancer development improve, new therapeutic targets and treatment modalities will be initiated for all stages of the disease.

Further reading

Heidenreich A, Bolla M, Joniau S et al. *European Association of Urology Guidelines on Prostate Cancer* 2010.

National Institute for Health and Clinical Excellence. *CG58. Prostate Cancer: Diagnosis and Treatment* 2008.

CHAPTER 9

Bladder Cancer

Pippa Sangster and Alan Thompson

OVERVIEW

- Bladder cancer is the seventh most common overall cancer in the UK, with men more commonly diagnosed (5:2)
- Exposure to smoking and aromatic amines increases risk
- The most common presentation is frank haematuria
- Diagnosis is by urine dipstick, cytology, cystoscopy and upper tract imaging
- Over 90% of bladder cancers are transitional cell carcinoma
- At diagnosis 80–85% are superficial cancers
- Most superficial tumours are managed endoscopically and with intravesical therapies
- Approximately 70% of superficial tumours are recurrent
- Approximately 15% of superficial tumours progress
- At diagnosis 15–20% are muscle invasive
- Muscle invasive tumours require radical treatment with cystectomy or radiotherapy
- Neo-adjuvant chemotherapy has a proven survival advantage in muscle invasive disease

---

Introduction and epidemiology

Bladder cancer is frequently diagnosed within the UK, with 10,091 new cases identified in 2007. It is the most common tumour of the urinary system and accounts for around 1 in every 29 new cases of cancer each year in the UK, with a male:female ratio of 5:2. In females it is the eleventh most common cancer, whilst in males it is the fourth most common. It is generally a disease of the older population with 80% of new cases diagnosed in patients over 65 years old.

Bladder cancer is the eighth most common cause of cancer deaths within the UK; however, the survival rates have improved dramatically over the past 30 years. Approximately half of patients diagnosed are likely to survive for at least 10 years and survival rates are higher for patients who have been diagnosed at a younger age.

ABC of Urology, Third Edition.
Edited by Chris Dawson and Janine M. Nethercliffe.
© 2012 John Wiley & Sons, Ltd. Published 2012 by John Wiley & Sons, Ltd.

- 57% of men survive > 5 years
- 47% of women survive > 5 years

The biggest risk factor is smoking, which has been shown to triple the risk of developing bladder cancer, as well as increasing long-term mortality rates. Passive smoking in children can increase their lifetime risk by 40%.

There are also a number of occupational exposures that are thought to be related to bladder cancer. Most common amongst these are the aromatic amines, which are found in the printing, hairdressing, iron and aluminium processing, industrial painting, and gas and tar manufacturing industries.

Presentation

Eighty per cent of patients with bladder cancer will present with painless visible haematuria. Other symptoms include dysuria, urgency and bladder pain, although these are less likely to be seen in superficial bladder cancer. Painful haematuria is a worrying sign, as pronounced irritative symptoms may indicate muscle-invasive disease or carcinoma *in situ* (CIS). Loin pain may be a sign of ureteric obstruction, but together with a pelvic mass or cachexia these signs and symptoms are very rare.

The guidelines for referral to a haematuria clinic are dealt with in chapter 2.

Investigation

Urine dipsticks

Haematuria can be microscopic (non-visible – seen only on urinalysis or light microscopy) or macroscopic (visible). Whilst the sensitivity of urine dipsticks may vary from one manufacturer to another, significant haematuria is considered to be 1+ or greater. Trace haematuria should be considered negative. Haematuria is defined as >3 RBC/high power field (hpf) of centrifuged sediment under the microscope. A positive test on a urine dipstick can indicate haematuria, haemoglobinuria or myoglobinuria. The reagent sticks work by detecting a change in the chromogen by the peroxidase activity of haemoglobin with the degree of colour change directly related to the amount of red blood cells (RBCs) present (Figure 1.1, Chapter 1).

False positive readings can be seen when there is contamination with menstrual blood, with dehydration (which concentrates the number of RBCs produced) and with exercise. If the testing is done near bleach and cleaning agents containing hydrogen peroxides, this can also lead to a false positive result.

Midstream urine (MSU)

Haematuria in the presence of infection is common. Once the infection has been treated, a dipstick should be repeated to confirm the post-treatment absence of haematuria. A urinary tract infection (regardless of haematuria) can be the first presentation of significant genito-urinary pathology, and should be further investigated if clinically indicated.

Infection is most readily excluded by a negative dipstick result for both leucocytes and nitrites. Otherwise an MSU negative for pyuria and culture are required.

Urine cytology

This should ideally be performed on a mid-morning stream and include the whole voided volume. Samples must be processed without delay. Although it is a useful investigation in the management of urothelial carcinoma, a negative test does not rule out malignancy. This test lacks sensitivity for the low-grade superficial tumours that constitute the majority of transitional cell carcinomas. Most reported sensitivities for low-grade tumours are in the region of 10–30%, whereas in high-grade tumours sensitivities are as high as 90%. Despite high specificity, it is not possible to localise cancer based on urine cytology alone. Therefore, a positive test result always needs further investigations.

Reactive changes secondary to infection, stone, previous instrumentation and intravesical therapy may lead to a false positive result.

There are other urinary biomarkers available such as NMP22/BTA/telomerase. In general, these new markers give a higher sensitivity than urinary cytology, but their specificity is usually lower. These markers are expensive and as they are not yet superior enough to replace cystoscopy, they remain an unnecessary expense.

Imaging

All patients with microscopic haematuria should undergo a plain film x-ray and a renal ultrasound scan to detect stones, renal masses, hydronephrosis and possibly filling defects within the bladder. Patients with frank haematuria may go on to further imaging depending on the result of the cystoscopy. Intravenous urography (IVU) can be used to detect filling defects in the calyces, renal pelvis and ureters, and hydronephrosis, but many hospitals are now routinely using computed tomography (CT) urograms as an alternative. CT urography has the disadvantage of a higher radiation exposure than IVU, and depending on the centre, both availability and cost can limit its use (see Figure 9.1).

Cystoscopy

This is a procedure usually performed by a urologist that allows visual access to the urethra, prostate, bladder neck and bladder. It

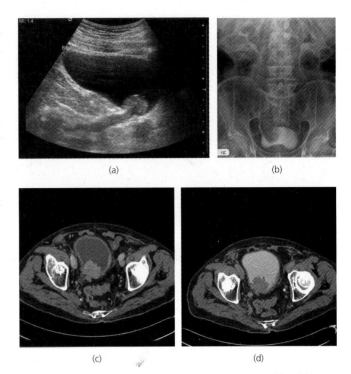

(a)   (b)

(c)   (d)

Figure 9.1 Filling defects in bladder seen on (a) U/S; (b) IVU; (c) and (d) CT.

is generally performed under local anaesthetic and the procedure takes approximately two minutes to carry out. A flexible cystoscope (see Figure 9.2) is inserted into the bladder through the urethra and at the same time the bladder is filled with saline to improve the view of the bladder wall. As the bladder fills, the patient may experience an uncomfortable urge to urinate. If an abnormality is detected the patient will require a general anaesthetic to undergo biopsy or resection of a lesion with a larger rigid cystoscope.

Fluorescence cystoscopy

This is an advanced form of cystoscopy, also known as photodynamic diagnosis (PDD), which involves instilling a chemical (5-aminolevulinic acid or its hexyl-ester Hexvix) within the bladder with a catheter prior to cystoscopy. The photochemical is metabolised in all cells to haem, a non-fluorescent product. However, in tumour cells protoporphyrin IX (fluorescent in blue light) accumulates probably due to iron deficiency. An intense blue light shone during the time of cystoscopy produces a red fluorescence,

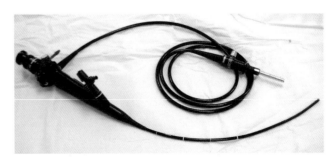

Figure 9.2 Flexible cytoscope.

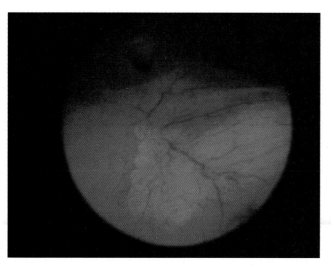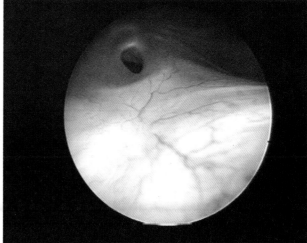

Figure 9.3 CIS of the bladder visualised with fluorescent cystoscopy (left) and standard cystoscopy.

which may result in higher tumour detection rates than the normal white light cystoscopy. Several studies have shown that PDD increases the detection rate of bladder tumours (particularly CIS) and thus improves resection, resulting in fewer early recurrences although it does not alter progression rates. However, the low specificity of PDD remains a problem.

The European Association of Urology now recommends its use for the diagnosis of CIS (Figure 9.3).

There is also an increased pick-up rate when cystoscopy is performed using narrow band imaging.

Classification and staging

Over 90% of bladder cancers are transitional cell carcinoma (TCC). The remaining 5–10% comprise squamous cell carcinoma, adenocarcinoma, sarcoma, small cell carcinoma and secondary deposits from cancers elsewhere in the body.

The 2009 TNM classification approved by the Union Internationale Contre le Cancer (UICC) has been widely accepted. Approximately 75–85% of patients with bladder cancer present with disease confined to the mucosa (stage Ta, CIS) or submucosa (stage T1).

The most significant prognostic factors for bladder cancer are grade, depth of invasion and the presence of CIS (Box 9.1 and Figure 9.4).

Most hospital pathologists are still using the 1973 World Health Organization classification, which divides cancers into three grades (G1 to G3) depending on how well differentiated they are.

Grade 1: well differentiated
Grade 2: moderately differentiated
Grade 3: poorly differentiated

Treatment

Superficial bladder cancer (Ta, T1 and CIS)

This represents 70–80% of newly diagnosed bladder cancers (see Figure 9.5). In most cases the risk of progression to distant disease

Box 9.1	**2009 TNM classification of urinary bladder cancer**
T	**Primary tumour**
TX	Primary tumour cannot be assessed
T0	No evidence of primary tumour
Ta	Non-invasive papillary carcinoma
Tis	Carcinoma *in situ*: 'flat tumour'
T1	Tumour invades subepithelial connective tissue
T2	Tumour invades muscle
	T2a Tumour invades superficial muscle (inner half)
	T2b Tumour invades deep muscle (outer half)
T3	Tumour invades perivesical tissue
	T3a Microscopically
	T3b Macroscopically (extravesical mass)
T4	Tumour invades any of the following: prostate, uterus, vagina, pelvic wall or abdominal wall
T4a	Tumour invades prostate, uterus or vagina
T4b	Tumour invades pelvic wall or abdominal wall
N	**Lymph nodes**
NX	Regional lymph nodes cannot be assessed
N0	No regional lymph node metastasis
N1	Metastasis in a single lymph node in the true pelvis (hypogastric, obturator, external iliac or presacral)
N2	Metastasis in multiple lymph nodes in the true pelvis (hypogastric, obturator, external iliac or presacral)
N3	Metastasis in a common iliac lymph node(s)
M	**Distant metastasis**
M0	No distant metastasis
M1	Distant metastasis

(*Source:* TNM Classification 2009)

is low. However, it is important to recognise those patients in whom the tumour is likely to progress. Therefore, management of superficial bladder cancer requires a long-term commitment and may mean lifelong follow-up if there are frequent recurrences, or where there is CIS. Superficial bladder cancers are a stage grouping of 3 distinct tumours (Ta, T1 and CIS) grouped together because they are managed in a similar way – endoscopically and with the

BLADDER CANCER STAGING (TNM)

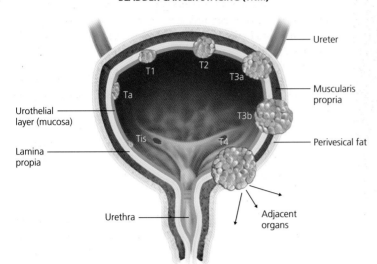

Figure 9.4 A schematic representation of the primary tumour stage of bladder cancer according to the TNM (2009).

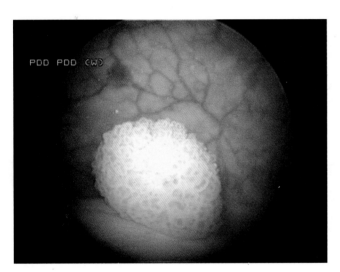

Figure 9.5 Cystoscopic view of superficial bladder cancer.

use of intravesical therapies. There is some controversy with this classification and there are certain subgroups within this category, namely carcinoma *in situ* (CIS) and G3pT1 tumours, which have a very high risk of progression.

Low-risk tumours (grade 1 or 2)

The aim of treatment in this group is to remove all visible tumours with a transurethral resection of bladder tumour (TURBT) as well as providing tissue with underlying detrusor muscle for correct pathological grading. This operation is performed under a general anaesthetic and generally requires a short hospital admission. Complications of this procedure include infection, haematuria, bladder perforation and urethral stricture.

If the tumour is completely resected in these low-risk tumours, only 30% of patients will go on to have early recurrence and 15% of these will be upstaged.

In addition to the surgical procedure, it is now recommended that all patients undergoing their first procedure should receive an intravesical dose of mitomycin C. A single postoperative dose within 24 hours of the surgery has been shown to decrease the relative risk of bladder cancer recurrence by 39%.

Some of these apparently low-risk patients may exhibit persistent multifocal disease that requires frequent admissions to hospital for further surgical procedures. They can be offered a further 6-weekly course of further intravesical chemotherapy.

Cystoscopic follow-up of patients is tailored to the risk category of the tumour. Low-risk patients initially have a cystoscopy at 3 months and if no tumour is seen, repeat cystoscopy occurs at 9 months and then yearly for 5 years. Higher risk tumours will require longer cystoscopic follow-up (see below).

High-risk tumours (CIS or grade 3)

Patients may require an early second TURBT when the initial resection was incomplete or if a high-grade, non-muscle invasive tumour has been reported by the pathologist.

These high-risk patients are at significant risk of both recurrence and upstaging of their disease. They may be offered adjuvant treatment with intravesical Bacillus Calmette-Guerin (BCG) in an attempt to preserve the bladder, or be considered for early primary cystectomy. It is thought that BCG attaches onto the urothelium of the bladder and mediates an immune response that decreases the rate of recurrence and possibly progression of the bladder cancer. Initially it is instilled into the bladder weekly. The BCG is retained within the bladder for two hours each time. This process is repeated for a total of six weeks. This is then repeated at 3-monthly and then 6-monthly intervals for three years with regular cystoscopic surveillance to ensure there is no progression.

BCG failure, described as an increasing number of recurrences, higher grade/stage or the appearance of CIS, is an indication to proceed to cystectomy.

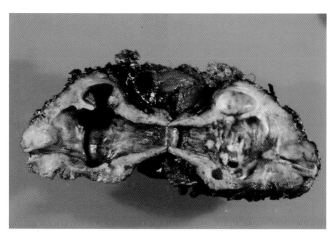

Figure 9.6 Macroscopic picture of cystectomy specimen (courtesy of Charles Jameson).

There is no role for radiotherapy in the management of high-risk superficial bladder cancer

Muscle invasive bladder cancer

Between 15 and 20% of bladder cancers are muscle invasive at the time of presentation. Initial management includes TURBT of the exophytic lesion to establish the diagnosis. A careful bimanual examination under the same anaesthetic must be performed to help with treatment decisions. A CT scan of chest, abdomen and pelvis should be performed to complete staging. A bone scan may be indicated if there is suspicion of bone metastases.

Historically the gold standard was to recommend immediate cystectomy in fit patients with muscle invasive bladder cancer and to reserve radiotherapy for those patients either too old or too unfit to undergo surgery. However, patients should be offered one of three options for control of the disease in their bladder as there is no current evidence that any one option is superior to any of the other options in terms of survival. After appropriate counselling, and discussion with both surgical and non-surgical oncologist, patients may be offered:

1 Cystectomy with or without some form of orthotopic bladder reconstruction (replacement bladder fashioned from bowel) (see Figure 9.6)
2 External beam radiotherapy
3 Selective bladder preservation whereupon the decision to either remove or irradiate the bladder is made dependent upon the response to neo-adjuvant chemotherapy.

Neo-adjuvant chemotherapy, usually with gemcitabine and cis-platin, has been shown in an individual patient data meta-analysis of randomised studies to confer a significant survival benefit, and should be offered to all patients with muscle invasive disease.

Further reading

European Association Urology Guidelines. http://www.uroweb.org/.
British Association of Urological Surgeons. http://www.baus.org.uk/.
Office for National Statistics, 2010 Cancer Statistics registrations. Registrations of cancer diagnosed in 2007, England.
Denzinger S, Wieland WF, Otto W, Filbeck T, Knuechel R, Burger M. Does photodynamic transurethral resection of bladder tumour improve the outcome of initial T1 high-grade bladder cancer? A long-term follow-up of a randomized study. *BJU Int* 2008 Mar; 101(5): 566–9. Epub 2007 Nov 5.
Sylvester RJ et al. (2004) A single immediate postoperative instillation of chemotherapy decreases the risk of recurrence in patients with stage Ta T1 bladder cancer: a meta-analysis of published results of randomized clinical trials. *J Urol* 171: 2186–90.

CHAPTER 10

Renal Cancer

Esther McLarty, Jonathan Aning and Simon J. Freeman

OVERVIEW

- Renal cell cancer accounts for 2% of all cancers diagnosed worldwide and the majority of renal malignancies
- The incidence of renal cell cancer is rising; increasing use of cross-sectional imaging is contributing to the rise because more small, low-stage, asymptomatic renal cell cancers are being diagnosed
- Surgery is the only evidence-based curative therapy for patients with localised disease. Where indicated partial nephrectomy should be considered
- A new generation of targeted medical therapies has increased the survival of patients with metastatic disease and the applications of these treatments will continue to evolve
- Transitional cell carcinoma of the renal pelvis and ureter is rare and has similar risk factors to those of bladder cancer

Introduction

Renal cancers are relatively rare but potentially lethal urological malignancies. Eighty-five per cent of renal cancers are adenocarcinomas or renal cell carcinomas (RCC), arising from tubular cells in the renal parenchyma (see Figure 10.1). Tumours arising from the urothelium of the renal pelvis and ureter make up most of the remainder of renal malignancies (10%) and are termed transitional cell carcinomas (TCC).

Epidemiology

RCC accounts for 2% of all cancers diagnosed worldwide. The incidence peaks at 60–70 years, with a male:female ratio of 1.5:1. Fifty per cent of patients with RCC will die from their condition and 25% of patients have metastases at presentation.

The incidence of RCC in the UK is rising with over 6000 cases diagnosed annually. Increasing use of cross-sectional imaging in the investigation of unrelated conditions has led to an increase

in the diagnosis of small, asymptomatic renal masses that might otherwise have remained undiagnosed.

Aetiology

The majority of RCCs (98%) are sporadic, and 2% occur in individuals with an inherited genetic predisposition. Studies of patients with a family history of RCC have led to major advances in our understanding of RCC tumour genesis.

Environmental factors

Renal cell carcinoma is prevalent in developed countries. Population studies have identified that risk factors associated with RCC are smoking, obesity and low socio-economic status. Migrants to Western societies from low incidence populations may adopt an increased risk of RCC. Nutrition is acknowledged to play an important role in risk reduction: fruit, vegetables, alcohol in moderation and certain vitamins have all been demonstrated to be protective.

Anatomical factors

Congenital and acquired abnormalities of anatomy, for example horseshoe kidneys and acquired cystic kidney, are associated with an increased risk of RCC.

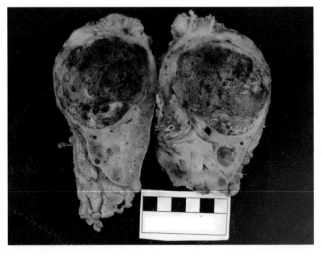

Figure 10.1 Tumour in upper pole of kidney.

Table 10.1 Characteristic features of Von Hippel-Lindau disease.

Features of Von Hippel-Lindau
Hypervascular tumours of the central nervous system and retina
Phaeochromocytomas
Pancreatic cysts
Pancreatic islet cell tumours
Epididymal cystadenomas
Endolymphatic sac tumours

Medical factors

Hypertension is associated with an increased risk of renal cancer. Patients undergoing dialysis have a 3–4-fold increased risk of RCC. Immunosuppressed transplant patients are also acknowledged to be at increased risk for RCC in their non-transplanted kidney. There is no conclusive evidence to date to indicate that urinary tract infections and kidney stones predispose patients to renal tumours.

Genetic factors

A number of rare genetic conditions predispose their sufferers to substantial increased risk of renal tumours. Often these renal tumours are of early onset, multifocal or bilateral.

Von Hippel-Lindau (VHL) syndrome is an autosomal dominantly inherited disease, affecting approximately 1 in 36 000 live births, characterised by the features listed in Table 10.1. VHL occurs due to the loss of both copies of the tumour suppressor gene at 3p25–26. This results in up-regulation of vascular endothelial growth factor (VEGF), the key angiogenic factor in RCC. Affected individuals have a 50% chance of developing RCC. The renal tumours are always clear cell type. Relatives of VHL patients should be offered genetic counselling and testing and enrolled in clinical monitoring programmes.

Hereditary papillary renal cell cancer is an autosomal dominantly inherited condition characterised by development of multiple RCCs of papillary variant. A mutation occurs in the c-MET proto-oncogene that regulates tyrosine kinase growth factors, which are responsible for epithelial proliferation and differentiation.

Familial clear cell renal cancer describes families with high risk of clear cell RCC but the molecular mechanisms underlying this are not understood.

Other familial RCC syndromes include hereditary leimyomatosis RCC, Burt-Hogg-Dubé syndrome, tuberous sclerosis and hyperparathyroidism jaw tumour.

Clinical features

Patients now rarely present with the classic triad of loin pain, haematuria and flank mass. More than 50% of RCCs are detected incidentally on abdominal imaging to investigate unrelated symptoms.

A full medical history should enquire about fatigue, weight loss, pyrexia and symptoms resulting from paraneoplastic syndromes listed in Table 10.2.

Abdominal examination may elicit a palpable mass and cervical lymphadenopathy. An acute left varicocele secondary to the

Table 10.2 Common paraneoplastic syndromes associated with renal cell cancer (RCC).

Paraneoplastic syndrome associated with RCC	Cause
Hypertension	Ectopic secretion of renin
Hypercalcaemia	Ectopic secretion of parathyroid hormone-like substance
Anaemia	Haematuria, chronic disease
Polycythaemia	Ectopic secretion of erythropoietin
Stauffer's syndrome (abnormal liver function tests, white blood cell loss, fever, areas of hepatic necrosis)	Unknown: resolves in most patients after nephrectomy

obstruction of the left testicular vein by tumour within the left renal vein may be present. In advanced disease lower limb oedema and a caput medusae (resulting from venous obstruction with tumour) may be observed.

Investigations

Venous blood samples should include full blood count, urea, creatinine, calcium, liver function tests and erythrocyte sedimentation rate. A blood pressure measurement is mandatory.

Radiological investigations are fundamental in renal cancer diagnosis and disease staging. Ultrasound may distinguish between cystic, solid and complex renal lesions. Complex cysts seen on ultrasound should be further investigated with computed tomography and classified according to the Bosniak classification. Bosniak I or II cysts may be safely ignored. Bosniak IIF cysts will require ongoing radiological surveillance whilst Bosniak III or IV cysts require surgical exploration and/or removal (see Box 10.1).

Box 10.1 Bosniak classification

Bosniak I – Simple benign cyst with a hairline thin wall. No septa, calcification or solid components. Measures as water density on CT and does not enhance with contrast material

Bosniak II – A benign cyst that may contain a few hairline thin septa. May show fine calcification. Uniformly high-attenuation lesions less than 3 cm that are sharply marginated and do not enhance

Bosniak IIF – Cysts contain more hairline thin septa than Bosniak II cysts. May show minimal enhancement of a hairline thin septum or may be thickening of septa or wall. May contain calcification. No enhancement with contrast. No enhancing soft tissue elements

Bosniak III – Indeterminate cystic masses that have thickened irregular walls or septa in which enhancement can be seen

Bosniak IV – Clearly malignant cystic lesions that contain enhancing soft tissue components

---

Contrast enhanced computed tomography (CT) of the chest and abdomen is the gold standard to stage renal tumours (see Figure 10.2). Hounsfield units measure the degree of enhancement when the kidney is viewed in pre- and post-contrast phases. A renal malignancy should enhance a minimum change of 20 Hounsfield units. Magnetic resonance imaging (MRI) and Doppler ultrasound

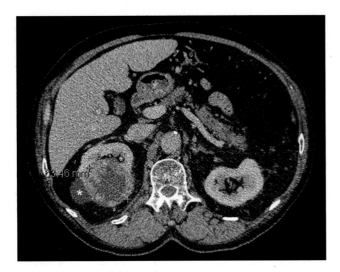

Figure 10.2 CT scan of right renal tumour.

are useful in determining invasion in the renal vein or inferior cava. MRI may be used to evaluate renal lesions when the use of nephrotoxic contrast agents is contraindicated. Isotope renography may assess differential kidney function if renal function is compromised to guide management regarding postoperative renal function or the need for nephron sparing surgery. Once identified and radiologically staged a renal tumour can be classified as localised, locally advanced or metastatic.

It is important to note that radiological imaging is not 100% diagnostic of renal lesions. Histological analysis is the only way to confirm a diagnosis. Consequently 5–10% of suspected renal malignancies removed surgically will prove to be benign. It is accepted that the potential harm of leaving an abnormal lesion in situ outweighs the risks from excision of a benign lesion. Preoperative radiologically guided renal biopsy has to date proved unreliable in differentiating malignant and benign lesions.

Staging by the TNM classification (Table 10.3), once histological confirmation has been obtained, is the most important prognostic indicator for RCC.

Treatment

Small renal lesions

Surveillance of localised renal lesions less than 4 cm in diameter with radiological imaging alone may be appropriate. Incidental tumours identified in the elderly or patients with significant co-morbidities may be watched because they are unlikely to cause morbidity or mortality earlier than the patient's pre-existing medical condition. Intervention can be considered where fast growing renal lesions are evident on serial imaging, or symptoms develop.

Surgery is the gold standard treatment for localised renal cancer. Radical nephrectomy (removal of the whole kidney, covered in Gerota's fascia) or partial nephrectomy (removal of part of the kidney) may be performed using a variety of techniques. The complications of surgery are illustrated in Box 10.2.

Laparoscopic radical nephrectomy is now widely practised and is accepted to be the gold standard treatment for T1 tumours less

Table 10.3 The 2009 TNM staging of renal cell cancer.

T	Primary tumour
Tx	Primary tumour cannot be assessed
T0	No evidence of primary tumour
T1	Tumour ≤ 7 cm in greatest dimension, limited to the kidney
T1a	Tumour ≤ 4 cm in greatest dimension, limited to the kidney
T1b	Tumour >4 cm but ≤ 7 cm in greatest dimension
T2	Tumour >7 cm in greatest dimension, limited to the kidney
T2a	Tumour >7 cm but ≤ 10 cm in greatest dimension
T2b	Tumour >10 cm limited to the kidney
T3	Tumour extends into major veins or directly invades adrenal gland or perinephric tissues but not into the ipsilateral adrenal gland and not beyond Gerota's fascia
T3a	Tumour grossly extends into the renal vein or its segmental (muscle-containing) branches or tumour invades perirenal and/or renal sinus (peripelvic) fat but not beyond Gerota's fascia
T3b	Tumour grossly extends into the vena cava below the diaphragm
T3c	Tumour grossly extends into the vena cava above the diaphragm or invades the wall of the vena cava
T4	Tumour invades beyond Gerota's fascia (including contiguous extension into the ipsilateral adrenal gland)
N	**Lymph nodes**
Nx	Regional lymph nodes cannot be assessed
N0	No regional lymph node metastasis
N1	Metastasis in a single regional lymph node
N2	Metastasis in more than one regional lymph node
M	**Distant metastasis**
M0	No distant metastasis
M1	Distant metastasis

(*Source:* TNM Classification 2009).

Box 10.2 **Complications of nephrectomy**

Complications of nephrectomy
Injury to gastrointestinal organs – spleen, liver, pancreas, bowel
Bleeding from major blood vessels – renal artery, renal vein, inferior vena cava, aorta
Pleural injury – pneumothorax
Ileus
Renal failure
Early or late infection – urinary tract, lower respiratory tract, wound
Systemic complications – pulmonary embolus (tumour thrombus/clot), deep vein thrombosis, myocardial infarction, death
Incisional hernia

---

than 7 cm in diameter. Larger tumours may be considered suitable for minimally invasive surgery dependent on surgeon ability, and technical difficulty may lead a surgeon to convert to an open surgical procedure. New approaches to nephrectomy are constantly being pioneered: single port laparoscopic, robotic, and natural orifice transluminal surgery are current concepts. The advantages of minimally invasive techniques over open surgery are accelerated patient recovery and return to function; however, this must be achieved without oncological compromise.

Partial nephrectomy may be performed in suitable patients by a laparoscopic or open approach. Absolute and relative indications are listed in Box 10.3. The kidney is mobilised, the renal tumour identified and the arterial supply clamped or controlled, whilst the abnormal lesion is removed under direct vision. In complex open surgery, the kidney may be cooled by ice prior to clamping to reduce the negative effects of ischaemia. The surgical margin must be clear of tumour; depth of margin does not affect risk of local recurrence. If there is any evidence of oncological compromise a radical nephrectomy is performed.

Box 10.3 **Indications for performing partial nephrectomy**

Indications for partial nephrectomy in patients with renal cell cancer

Absolute – Tumour in a solitary functioning kidney
Relative – Multifocal or bilateral renal tumours or chronic renal insufficiency
Elective – Tumours less than 7 cm, away from the pelvicalyceal system, in patients with a normal contralateral kidney

(*Source:* TNM Classification 2009)

Cryo-surgery and radiofrequency ablation of renal lesions less than 4 cm in size are experimental minimally invasive treatments that have demonstrated promise. The results of large scale randomised controlled trials to confirm their utilities are awaited.

Large renal lesions

Open radical nephrectomy is now reserved for the removal of large tumours over 7 cm in diameter with or without evidence of ipsilateral adrenal or nodal tumour involvement. This may be performed via a loin, abdominal or thoraco-abdominal incision. Tumours with renal vein or inferior vena cava involvement may be amenable to surgery and may require cardiac bypass during the procedure.

Metastatic disease

Patients with metastatic disease have a poor prognosis. In some patients, with either single organ site metastasis or solitary metastasis and good performance status, attempted curative surgery in the form of radical nephrectomy and metasectomy may be curative.

Immunotherapy (interleukin and interferon) has been superseded as first-line treatment by a new generation of targeted therapies, which act by blocking angiogenesis pathways. Sporadic RCCs have been demonstrated to develop and progress because they over-express factors that promote angiogenesis. Thus targeted drugs aim to slow or arrest tumour growth in responsive patients. Randomised controlled trials indicate that Tyrosine Kinase Inhibitors (Sunitinib and Sorafenib) and mammalian target of rapamycin inhibitors (Temsirolimus and Everolimus) prolong progression-free survival in patients with metastatic RCC by 3–6 months. These agents are used in current clinical practice. Novel targeted therapies, their ability to work in synergy, in addition to in combination with, cytoreductive nephrectomy (removing the primary tumour in the presence of known metastases) are under investigation.

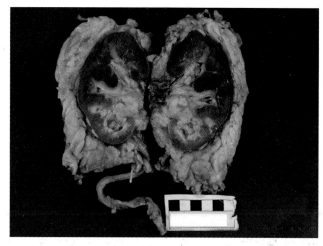

Figure 10.3 Transitional Cell Carcinoma of the renal pelvis. The transitional cell carcinoma is seen arising from the lower part of the renal pelvis.

Radiotherapy has a role mainly limited to palliation of painful bone metastases and RCCs are not sensitive to traditional chemotherapeutic agents.

Transitional cell carcinoma (TCC) of the renal pelvis and ureters

TCC of the renal pelvis and ureter are rare and the risk factors are similar to TCC of the bladder (described in Chapter 9) (Figure 10.3). The majority present with painless, visible haematuria. Some patients may suffer 'clot colic' (loin pain caused by the passage of clots down the ureter) and a minority will be picked up during investigation of a synchronous bladder TCC. Diagnosis is usually made on a computed tomography urogram or intravenous urogram by identification of a filling defect. Selective ureteric cytology, retrograde pyelography and ureteroscopic biopsy may be used to confirm the diagnosis. Staging according to the TNM classification is performed by CT.

Laparoscopic or open radical nephro-ureterectomy (removal of the kidney and entire ureter) is the gold standard treatment for non-metastatic disease. In patients with a single functioning kidney, bilateral disease or multiple co-morbidities: percutaneous or ureteroscopic tumour ablation and installation of topical chemotherapy are minimally invasive, nephron sparing therapeutic options. Palliative chemotherapy may be considered in patients with advanced or metastatic disease.

Further reading

Ljungberg B, Cowan N, Hanbury DC, Hora M, Kuczyk MA, Merseburger AS et al. European Association of Urology. *2010 Guidelines on Renal Cell Carcinoma*. Available online at http://www.uroweb.org/gls/pdf/Renal%20Cell%20Carcinoma%202010.pdf (last accessed November 2010).
Mundy AR, Fitzpatrick JM, Neal DE, George NJR (eds). *The Scientific Basis of Urology*. London, Informa Healthcare, 2010.

CHAPTER 11

Testicular Tumours

Jessica Wrigley, Anne Y. Warren and Danish Mazhar

OVERVIEW

- More than 95% of testicular tumours are germ cell tumours (GCT)
- GCTs need expert treatment and advanced disease is treated in specialist centres
- GCTs are very sensitive to cisplatin-based chemotherapy and the prognosis is good, even with the majority of cases of advanced disease
- Over 90% of GCTs are cured

Table 11.1 Clinical characteristics of seminoma vs. non-seminomatous germ cell tumours.

	Seminoma	Non-Seminoma
Tumour markers	AFP not raised HCG raised in ~20%	AFP and/or HCG raised in ~75%
Tumour behaviour	Less aggressive Radiosensitive	More aggressive with shorter tumour doubling time Less radiosensitive
Mean age at diagnosis	30–40	20–30
Timing of relapse	Potential to relapse late (sometimes >10 yrs)	~95% of relapses occur in the first 2 yrs

Introduction

Over 95% of testicular cancers are germ cell tumours, of which approximately 60% are seminomas and approximately 40% are non-seminomas. Non-germ cell tumours of the testis are uncommon and include Leydig cell tumours, Sertoli cell tumours and lymphomas.

Male testicular germ cell tumours (TGCTs) are the most common neoplasms in males aged 15–44 years although overall they remain relatively rare, with an incidence of around 6 per 100 000 population in the UK. In men, germ cell cancers account for around 1% of all malignancies and 0.1% of male cancer-related mortality.

Germ cell tumours (GCTs) are a heterogeneous group of neoplasms, and it is postulated that they arise during fetal development. They originate mainly in the gonads and more rarely from extragonadal sites along the midline including the retroperitoneum, sacrum, mediastinum and pineal gland. This pattern of distribution reflects the route of migratory primordial germ cells to the genital ridge.

In the testis, the presence of atypical germ cells lining the seminiferous tubules is known as intratubular germ cell neoplasia (ITGCN). This represents pre-invasive disease and is a risk factor for development of a malignant germ cell tumour which is characterised by growth outside the confines of the basement membranes into the testicular interstitium. Lymphatic spread is the most common cause of metastasis, occurring via spermatic cord lymphatics to the retroperitoneal lymph node chain. Haematogenous invasion leads to extranodal distant metastases to sites such as the lung, liver, bone and brain.

Histological classification of TGCTs

Germ cell tumours can be broadly divided into two classes with different clinical characteristics (Table 11.1):

1 Seminomas (see Figure 11.1)
2 Non-seminomatous germ cell tumours (NSGCT) (see Figures 11.2 and 11.3).

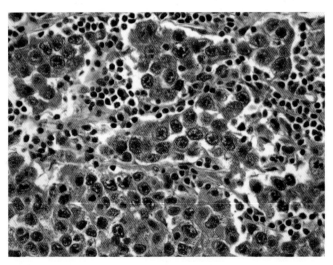

Figure 11.1 Histological appearance of seminoma.

ABC of Urology, Third Edition.
Edited by Chris Dawson and Janine M. Nethercliffe.
© 2012 John Wiley & Sons, Ltd. Published 2012 by John Wiley & Sons, Ltd.

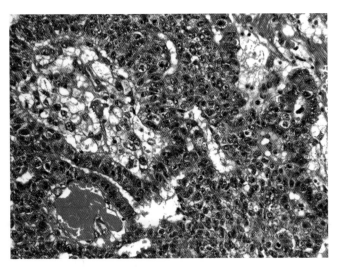

Figure 11.2 Histological appearance of embryonal carcinoma.

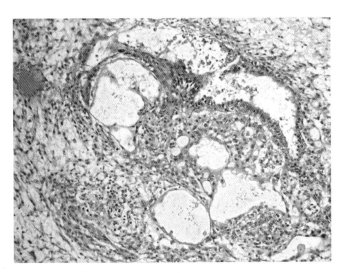

Figure 11.3 Histological appearance of yolk sac tumour.

The WHO classification system subdivides these according to histopathological features. Of note, less than 50% of malignant testicular germ cell tumours are composed of a single cell type, i.e. 'pure' type, the majority being classified as 'mixed' tumours.

Clinical assessment

Presenting symptoms/signs

- ~ 90 % of patients have a lump
- 31% have pain
- 29% describe a dragging sensation
- 15% have inflammation
- 10% give a history of trauma
- <5% have gynaecomastia
- 2% have bilateral tumours

In a small minority of patients, the primary tumour manifestation is extragonadal, with patients presenting, for example, with persistent lower back pain due to large retroperitoneal nodes or breathlessness as a result of widespread pulmonary metastases.

History

When assessing the patient's history, risk factors for the development of testicular tumours should be addressed (see Table 11.2).

Examination

Examination of both testes is essential. A suspicious mass is one that is within the testis, and is firm and non-fluctuating. Palpation of the spermatic cord for thickness and mobility should be performed. The chest should be examined and the abdomen and lymph node regions (neck, supraclavicular, axillary and inguinal) palpated. Any suspicious lesion should be referred urgently to the urology department for advice using the appropriate 2-week-wait system.

Investigations

Mandatory investigations include serum tumour markers alphafetoprotein (AFP) and human chorionic gonadotrophin (HCG). These are important not only in the staging of advanced germ cell cancers but also in the monitoring of disease and the detection of

Table 11.2 Risk factors for the development of testicular germ cell tumours.

Factor	Description
Family history	The two strongest associations with testis cancer are having a brother (relative risk 8) and having a father (relative risk 4) with a history of TGCT. A genetic component of TGCT is supported by demonstration of a higher risk to monozygotic twins of TGCT patients than to dizygotic twins and by the observation that the frequency of bilateral disease is higher among cases with a family history than those without
Cryptorchidism.	There is a well-established association between testicular maldescent and TGCTs. The increased risk is debatable (2–17-fold is quoted in the literature). There is suggestive evidence that early correction (prepuberty) will decrease the risk, though this remains controversial. The testis cancer risk applies to both testes and not only to the one affected by maldescent
Previous testicular cancer	Five per cent of patients with testicular tumours harbour intra-tubular germ cell neoplasia (ITGCN) or carcinoma-in-situ within the contralateral testis (see management of the contralateral testis)
Klinefelter's syndrome	Klinefelter's syndrome (47XXY) is associated with a higher incidence of germ cell tumours, particularly primary mediastinal germ cell tumours
Testicular atrophy	Can be secondary to trauma, hormones and viral orchitis
Environmental factors	There are studies suggesting an association with higher socio-economic class

Table 11.3 Royal Marsden Hospital staging system for testicular germ cell tumours.

Stage I	No evidence of disease outside the testis
IM	As above but with persistently raised tumour markers
Stage II	Infradiaphragmatic nodal involvement
IIA	Maximum diameter <2 cm
IIB	Maximum diameter 2–5 cm
IIC	Maximum diameter >5–10 cm
IID	Maximum diameter >10 cm
Stage III	Supra- and infradiaphragmatic nodal involvement
	Abdominal nodes A, B, C as above
	Mediastinal nodes M+
	Neck nodes N+
Stage IV	Extralymphatic metastases
	Abdominal nodes A, B, C, as above
	Mediastinal or neck nodes as for stage III
	Lungs:
	L1 <3 metastases
	L2 Multiple metastases <2 cm maximum diameter
	L3 Multiple metastases >2 cm in diameter
	Liver involvement H+
	Other sites specified

disease relapse. Lactate dehydrogenase (LDH) can be an important prognostic factor in advanced disease and should also be determined prior to treatment.

Ultrasound of the scrotum can be used to confirm the presence of a testicular tumour with almost 100% sensitivity. After radical orchidectomy, computerised tomography (CT), with oral and intravenous contrast, of the chest, abdomen and pelvis is required for radiological staging (Table 11.3). Bone scans should be obtained in patients with elevated levels of alkaline phosphatase or if bone metastases are clinically suspected. Imaging of the brain by CT or MRI is required in patients with clinical signs potentially indicating brain metastases, in patients with extensive lung and/or retroperitoneal disease, or if the tumour marker levels are very high.

Management (Figure 11.4)

Options post-orchidectomy for stage I seminoma include surveillance, adjuvant para-aortic node radiotherapy, and a single cycle of adjuvant carboplatin chemotherapy. For stage I non-seminoma the options are surveillance and adjuvant chemotherapy with 2 cycles of bleomycin, etoposide and cisplatin (BEP). Retroperitoneal lymph node dissection (RPLND) in this context is practised in some countries. For metastatic germ cell cancer, the management is usually with 3 or 4 cycles of BEP (depending on prognostic grouping, see Table 11.4). Stage IIA or B seminoma can be treated with para-aortic radiotherapy.

Inguinal orchidectomy

All patients with testicular primary should have an orchidectomy. Radical orchidectomy is performed through an inguinal incision. The tumour-bearing testicle is resected along with the spermatic cord at the level of the internal inguinal ring. Complications include: infection, haemorrhage and possible reduced fertility (depending on the function of the remaining testis).

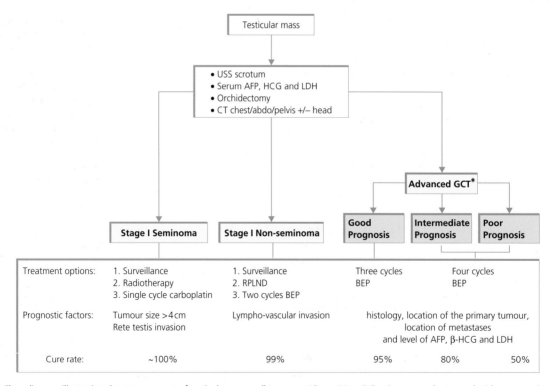

Figure 11.4 Flow diagram illustrating the management of testicular germ cell tumours. *Stage IIA or B Seminoma can be treated with para-aortic radiotherapy.

Table 11.4 International Germ Cell Consensus Classification Group prognostic grouping.

NSGCT	Seminoma
Good prognosis (92% 5-yr survival) with ALL of:	
Testis/retroperitoneal primary	Any primary site
No non-pulmonary visceral mets	No non-pulmonary visceral mets
AFP < 1000 ng/ml	Normal AFP
HCG < 5000 iu/l	Any HCG
LDH <1.5 upper limit normal	Any LDH
56% teratomas	90% seminomas
Intermediate prognosis (80% 5-yr survival) with ALL of:	
Testis/retroperitoneal primary	Any primary site
No non-pulmonary visceral mets	Non-pulmonary visceral mets
AFP ≥ 1000 and ≤ 10 000 ng/ml or	Normal AFP
HCG ≥ 5000 and ≤ 50 000 iu/l or	Any HCG
LDH ≥ 1.5 normal and ≤ 10 normal	Any LDH
28% teratomas	10% seminomas
Poor prognosis (48% 5-yr survival) with ANY of:	
Mediastinal primary or non-pulmonary visceral mets	
AFP > 10 000 ng/ml or	
HCG > 50 000 iu/l or	
LDH > 10 normal	
16% teratomas	

International Germ Cell Cancer Collaborative Group (IGCCCG). The International Germ Cell Classification: a prognostic factor-based staging system for metastatic germ cell cancer. *J. Clin Oncol.* 1997;15:594–603.

Stage I seminoma germ cell tumour (SGCT)

Following orchidectomy, the cure rate in stage I seminoma patients is almost 100% and can be achieved with any of three strategies:

1 Surveillance, with treatment on relapse,
2 Adjuvant chemotherapy with single-agent carboplatin, or
3 Adjuvant external beam radiotherapy to the para-aortic lymph nodes.

With surveillance alone, there is a 15–20% risk of disease relapse due to occult metastatic disease, but surveillance recognises that at least 80% of patients do not need any adjuvant treatment after orchidectomy and are therefore over-treated by adjuvant radiation or chemotherapy. Adjuvant chemotherapy with a single dose of carboplatin is equivalent in effectiveness to adjuvant radiotherapy; however, there is a trend towards the use of adjuvant chemotherapy due to the risk of secondary malignancy associated with external beam radiation. Short-term complications of carboplatin include myelosuppression, nausea and vomiting, fatigue and neurotoxicity.

Using tumour size >4 cm and rete testis invasion, patients with stage I seminoma can be subdivided into a low- and high-risk group of occult metastatic disease. Patients with *both* risk factors have a risk of occult disease of 32% and those with neither risk factor may have a relapse risk as low as 6%. Surveillance is an acceptable management strategy for both high- and low risk-patients, assuming they are compliant with the follow-up procedure.

Stage I non-seminoma germ cell tumour (NSGCT)

Following orchidectomy, the cure rate in stage I non-seminoma patients is 99% and can be achieved with any of three strategies:

1 Surveillance,
2 Adjuvant chemotherapy with 2 cycles of BEP (bleomycin, etoposide and cisplatin chemotherapy), or
3 Retroperitoneal lymph node dissection (RPLND).

In the case of surveillance, the relapse rate is 27–30%. Relapses occur in the retroperitoneum in 54–78% of patients and in the lungs in 13–31% of patients.

Vascular invasion (VI) of the primary tumour is the most important prognostic indicator for relapse. Patients with VI have a 48% risk of developing metastatic disease whereas only 14–22% of patients without VI will relapse. A risk adapted approach has been adopted in many centres with low-risk patients being managed with surveillance, and high-risk patients with 2 cycles of adjuvant BEP chemotherapy, which then reduces the relapse risk to 3%. Given the potential for long-term complications following BEP, however, (see below and Table 11.5), many clinicians favour surveillance in high-risk patients as well.

Complications of BEP chemotherapy include: myelosuppression, nausea and vomiting, fatigue, alopecia, hearing loss,

Table 11.5 Long-term complications of BEP chemotherapy.

Complication	Description
Bleomycin-related lung toxicity	Bleomycin lung is a radiological diagnosis. It progresses from pneumonitis to fibrosis and can be fatal. Risk factors include: age (especially >40 yrs), smoking and renal impairment
Treatment-related cardiovascular effects	There is emerging evidence to suggest that BEP chemotherapy and radiation may lead to a late excess risk of cardiovascular morbidity
Treatment-related secondary cancer	BEP chemotherapy and para-aortic radiation have been associated with an increased risk of second malignancies
Treatment-related infertility	Sperm banking prior to chemotherapy should be offered. Virtually all become oligospermic during BEP chemotherapy, but the majority recover sperm production, and can father children, usually without the use of cryopreserved semen
Cisplatin-related ototoxicity	Bilateral hearing deficits occur with cisplatin-based chemotherapy, but the deficits generally occur at sound frequencies of 4 kHz to 8 kHz, which is outside the range of conversational tones; therefore, hearing aids are rarely required if standard doses of cisplatin are administered

BEP = bleomycin, etoposide and cisplatin

bleomycin-induced pulmonary pneumonitis (in 10%) with potential to progress to fibrosis which can be fatal (1–2%), reduced fertility, and cardiovascular morbidity.

The role of primary nerve sparing retroperitoneal lymph node resection in stage I NSGCT is controversial and is rarely practised in the UK as the procedure is associated with significant morbidity, including: retrograde ejaculation in 6–8%, postoperative ascites and lymphocele development. Following surgery, relapses can still occur in around 10% of cases even when no microscopic disease is found at RPLND. Moreover, if significant disease is found in the resected lymph nodes, chemotherapy is then required.

Advanced germ cell tumours (stages II and III)

All testis-primary patients require orchidectomy, usually prior to chemotherapy, although some patients presenting with extensive metastatic disease should be treated urgently with primary chemotherapy first (with orchidectomy following later). Combination chemotherapy with BEP is the mainstay of treatment for advanced germ cell cancers. However, patients with stage IIA or B seminoma may be treated with para-aortic radiotherapy.

The histology, location of the primary tumour, location of metastases and serum levels of AFP, HCG and LDH are all used as prognostic markers to categorise patients into 'good', 'intermediate' and 'poor' prognostic groups (Table 11.4).

Good prognosis patients are treated with 3 cycles of BEP, and intermediate and poor prognosis patients with 4 cycles of BEP.

Non-seminoma patients with any residual masses >1 cm after chemotherapy should have the masses resected (if technically feasible) even if the tumour markers have normalised as they may contain viable tumour or mature teratoma as well as necrosis. If >10% of the resected tumour specimen contains viable cancer, or if the completeness of the resection is in doubt, consolidation chemotherapy may be justified. Post-chemotherapy residual masses in seminoma patients should not necessarily be resected and masses <3 cm can usually be followed with imaging. PET-CT may have a role in evaluating the nature of a residual mass in seminoma.

Management of the contralateral testis

Five per cent of patients with testicular tumours harbour intra-tubular germ cell neoplasia (ITGCN) or carcinoma-in-situ within the contralateral testis, detectable by open biopsy in 99% of cases. For patients with a testicular volume <12 ml and an age at diagnosis <30 years, the risk of TIGHT in the contralateral testis is >34% and biopsy is recommended. ITGCN can be treated with prophylactic orchidectomy or external beam radiotherapy to the testis as the risk of progression to an invasive malignancy is 70% at 5 years. Surveillance with testicular ultrasound is an option for those wishing to preserve fertility and avoid lifelong testosterone replacement, but if invasive cancer develops then orchidectomy will be required.

Patient follow-up

The aims of follow-up for patients with germ cell cancer include:

- detection of relapse (including late relapse)
- diagnosis of second cancers
- prevention, early diagnosis, and treatment of physical and psychological morbidity related to germ cell cancer or its therapy (Table 11.5).

Follow-up protocols are centre-specific but are generally highly structured and involve regular clinical examination (including examination of the contralateral testis), serum tumour markers, chest x-rays and CT scans. Patients on surveillance for stage I disease are CT scanned for two years for non-seminoma, and five years in seminoma (later recurrences are known to occur with seminoma).

Germ cell cancer is rare but curable, even if the initial presentation is with distant metastatic disease. It is important for patients who are on surveillance for stage I testicular germ cell cancer to rigorously attend follow-up assessments, as on recurrence the vast majority of men can be cured.

Further reading

Harland SJ, Cook PA, Fossa SD et al. Intratubular germ cell neoplasia of the contralateral testis in testicular cancer: defining a high risk group. *J Urol* 1998; 160: 1353–7.

Krege S, Beyer J, Souchon R et al. European Consensus Conference on Diagnosis and Treatment of Germ Cell Cancer: A Report of the Second Meeting of the European Germ Cell Cancer Consensus Group (EGCCCG): Part I. *Eur Urol* 2008; 53: 478–96.

Krege S, Beyer J, Souchon R et al. European Consensus Conference on Diagnosis and Treatment of Germ Cell Cancer: A Report of the Second Meeting of the European Germ Cell Cancer Consensus group (EGCCCG): Part II. *Eur Urol* 2008; 53: 497–513.

Classen J, Schmidberger H, Meisner C et al. Radiotherapy for stages IIA/B testicular seminoma: final report of a prospective multicenter clinical trial. *J Clin Oncol* 2003; 21: 1101–6.

Williams SD, Birch R, Einhorn LH, Irwin L, Greco FA, Lohrer PJ. Treatment of disseminated germ-cell tumors with cisplatin, bleomycin, and either vinblastine or etoposide, *N Engl J Med* 1987; 316: 1435–40.

CHAPTER 12

Urinary Tract Stone Disease

Farooq A. Khan

Prevalence of urinary stones

Urinary tract stone disease is relatively common in the UK with approximately 10% of the population suffering with a renal stone episode in their lifetime. Of these, half will go onto a further episode in the following 10 years. Certain risk factors for renal stone formation are recognised (Box 12.1). The common renal stone types are listed in Box 12.2.

Box 12.1 **Risk factors for stone formation**

- Male sex
- Age 20–50
- Geographical – more common in Northern Europe and hot climates (Middle East)
- Genetic – more common in Caucasians and Asians and less in African and US blacks
- Diet – high protein intake (Western diet)
- Occupation – sedentary workers at greater risk than manual workers
- Low fluid intake
- Drugs – steroids, chemotherapy for myeloproliferative disorders causes release of purines and uric acid

ABC of Urology, Third Edition.
Edited by Chris Dawson and Janine M. Nethercliffe.
© 2012 John Wiley & Sons, Ltd. Published 2012 by John Wiley & Sons, Ltd.

- Immobility – leads to bone demineralisation and raised urinary calcium levels
- Systemic disease – sarcoidosis
- Inflammatory bowel disease/malabsorptive states – cause high urinary oxalate levels (hyperoxaluria)
- Abnormal renal anatomy -- pelvi-ureteric junction obstruction and horseshoe kidney
- Family history – 25% of stone formers have a positive history

Box 12.2 **Stone types and composition**

Ninety per cent of all renal and ureteric stones are radiopaque.

- Calcium containing stones – 80% of all stones. Radiopaque
- Uric acid – 5–10%. Radiolucent
- Struvite (magnesium ammonium phosphate stones) – 10–15%. Can occupy the collecting system to form a staghorn calculus. Radiopaque
- Cystine – 1%. Faintly radiopaque. Occur only in cystinuria

Presentation and diagnosis of renal stones

Renal stones are often detected incidentally on imaging. They may also cause loin pain or haematuria – both microscopic (non-visible) or macroscopic (visible). Staghorn calculi can be a source of recurrent urinary tract infections (UTI) or more serious septic complications such as pyelonephritis, pus in the kidney (pyonephrosis) or perinephric abscess formation (see Figure 12.1).

Whilst 90% of renal stones are radiopaque and therefore visible on plain x-rays, small stones can be missed. Ultrasound has a high sensitivity in detecting renal stones (but not ureteric) and intravenous urography (IVU) delineates the location of stones within the kidney in a readily recognised x-ray format. However, the definitive imaging modality is non-contrast computed tomography (CT), which with 3-dimensional reconstruction can provide useful information for stone treatment planning (Figure 12.2; Box 12.3).

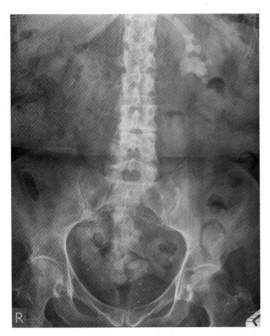

Figure 12.1 Left staghorn calculus seen on plain X-ray.

Box 12.3 **Advantages and disadvantages of non-contrast CT**

Advantages

- High sensitivity – 97%+
- Quick to perform
- Avoids use of intravenous contrast and possible contrast reactions and therefore can be used in renal failure
- Detects other causes of abdominal pain – ∼ 6–10% of cases initially thought to be ureteric colic

Disadvantages

- Higher radiation dose compared to short-series IVU
- Expensive – although little difference between IVU and CT in high volume units
- Not freely available in all units at all times
- Not easy to interpret compared to familiar IVU
- Sometimes difficult to distinguish between pelvic phleboliths and small distal ureteric stones

Management and treatment of renal stones

The management of renal stones depends on the size of the stone and its location in the kidney and the desire and need to be stone free.

Observation

Small, asymptomatic stones can be observed, especially those in elderly patients in whom stone progression is unlikely to affect them. However, whilst this is also reasonable in younger patients, small renal stones have a tendency to progress and become symptomatic requiring treatment. In general, stones greater than 4 mm will cause pain, progress or become symptomatic requiring treatment over a 3-year period in 20–50% of patients.

Extracorporeal shock wave lithotripsy (ESWL)

- ESWL uses shock waves directed under x-ray or ultrasound guidance onto the stone.
- Absorption of the shock wave energy fragments the stone allowing the fragments to be passed in the urine.
- ESWL is a useful modality in those patients who have stones less than 2 cm, are unfit for more extensive intervention with general anaesthesia, or after failure of endoscopic control.
- Success with ESWL is best seen in soft stones which are favourably located in the kidney allowing drainage of the fragments (not lower pole or those in a calyceal diverticulum).
- Success rates decline with increasing BMI and stone size and this treatment cannot be used in all patients (Box 12.4).

Endoscopic – flexible ureterorenoscopy

This is a very effective primary treatment for stones less than 2 cm or in those who have failed ESWL. It is suitable for:

- hard stones (cystine)
- lower pole stones
- patients who are obese and have skeletal abnormalities precluding safe tract formation in PCNL
- stones trapped in calyceal diverticula
- anatomically challenging kidneys such as a pelvic or horseshoe kidney.

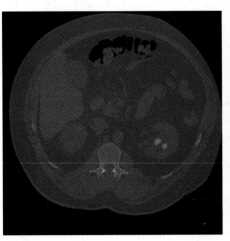

(a)

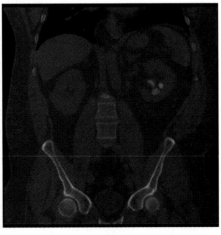

(b)

Figure 12.2 Large collection of stones seen on cross-section (a) and clearly defined on coronal CT as being in the lower pole and renal pelvis (b).

Flexible ureterorenoscopy can usually access the whole of the collecting system and can be used as an adjuvant treatment to PCNL to complete stone clearance. It can be safely used in anticoagulated patients.

Percutaneous nephrolithotomy (PCNL)

Under general anaesthesia and fluoroscopy a track is formed in the loin allowing a nephroscope to be passed directly into the collecting system and onto the stone(s). These are fragmented with an energy source (ultrasound, laser, pneumatic) and washed out. PCNL is an excellent treatment for large stones in excess of 2 cm and those located in the lower pole or trapped in a calyceal diverticulum. It is recommended treatment for staghorn calculi and can be combined with ESWL or flexible ureterorenoscopy to achieve a stone free status.

Laparoscopic surgery

Laparoscopy is rarely used but is increasing in popularity and provides excellent stone clearance rates with minimal morbidity and complications. Laparoscopic nephrectomy can be used for removing non-functioning kidneys (as a consequence of long-standing stone disease). Generally, function less than 15% is now recognised as the limit for preserving renal units in the presence of a normal contralateral kidney.

Open surgery

Open nephrolithotomy is not commonly performed but is useful for large renal stones where laparoscopic skill is not available or for staghorn calculi where a single treatment is the aim. Alternatively, once diminished renal function is confirmed on nuclear isotope studies (dimercapto succinic acid (DMSA) scan) a nephrectomy can be performed although nowadays the majority are undertaken laparoscopically.

Presentation and diagnosis of ureteric stones

Ureteric stones typically cause sudden severe colicky flank pain, radiating to the groin and genitalia resulting in a restless disposition as the patient attempts to find a comfortable position. Intense sensations of nausea and vomiting are common and the presence of macroscopic and more commonly microscopic haematuria is usual. Stones in the intramural ureter may additionally cause frequency and urgency as the stone irritates the trigone.

Beware of a leaking abdominal aortic aneurysm masquerading as ureteric colic in patients over the age of 60. Immediate imaging is recommended in this age group especially in the absence of documented haematuria.

Occasionally patients with a history of drug abuse will mimic the symptoms of renal or ureteric colic in order to obtain opiate analgesia

Investigation of acute ureteric colic

Acute ureteric colic is extremely painful, although ureteric stones can present with minimal pain. This highlights the point that the absence of pain does not mean that a stone has passed or serious ureteric obstruction is not present. Anti-emetics and intramuscular non-steroidal anti-inflammatory analgesia (ketoprofen) or rectally (diclofenac) are highly effective for the pain. Once this settles definitive imaging is required even if the pain completely subsides. Measurement of renal function (serum creatinine) and urinalysis should be undertaken in the emergency department. Absence of microscopic haematuria does not rule out the possibility of ureteric stone disease as its presence declines with the increasing interval between onset of symptoms and presentation. Clinical suspicion and judgement remain paramount in the diagnosis.

The absence of pain does not mean a stone has passed or that significant obstruction is not present. The location and size of the ureteric stone will determine whether this will pass spontaneously or require intervention. The smaller the stone and the lower this is in the ureter the more likely the stone will pass. Plain x-ray may identify ureteric stones but small stones may be easily missed especially overlying the bony pelvis (Figure 12.3).

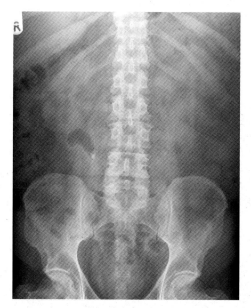

Figure 12.3 Radiopaque calculus seen in the mid ureter – just above the 4th right transverse process.

Non-contrast CT has in most units replaced an IVU as the definitive acute imaging modality given its greater sensitivity and specificity (97%+ and 95%+, respectively) (Box 12.3). IVUs are still used in some units and still have a role in certain stone treatment planning.

Management of ureteric stones

Conservative

Small stones that are less than 4 mm are likely to pass on their own accord (90%+) over the following weeks, further aided by the use of alpha-blockers, with the majority of 6 mm or less stones also spontaneously passed. Patients deemed unsuitable for conservative treatment include those with a stone greater than 7 mm, uncontrolled pain, prolonged obstruction that will result in irreversible nephron loss (usually obstruction lasting greater than two weeks), fever especially in the presence of obstruction, solitary kidneys, renal impairment or those who will be unable to work as a consequence of their stone.

Endoscopic

Stones that are large or have failed a trial of conservative treatment and are unlikely to pass, especially in the presence of ureteric obstruction, will need endoscopic extraction. Stones greater than 7 mm often require intervention. A ureteroscope is passed under general anaesthetic and the stone is fragmented with an energy source (often laser nowadays given its greater efficacy and safety profile in ureteric stone fragmentation). Occasionally, a stent is placed to relieve obstruction and pain prior to, or following, definitive stone treatment (see Figure 12.4).

ESWL

Stones in favourable locations and in the absence of obstruction can, where available, have shock wave treatment to fragment the

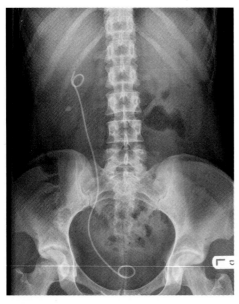

Figure 12.4 A ureteric stent was passed to unobstruct this ureter – and consequently resulted in the stone being pushed into the kidney. This was successfully treated by flexible ureterorenoscopy.

stone. Limited availability precludes its widespread use as a first-line treatment option for acute ureteric stones, with most urology units having to rely on a visiting lithotriptor every 2–4 weeks.

PCNL

PCNL is rarely used and usually only for large stones that are impacted in the upper ureter that have failed endoscopic fragmentation or are inaccessible due to a ureteric stricture.

Laparoscopic surgery

This is not used acutely but is an option in large stones in the upper ureter which are inaccessible endoscopically (laparoscopic ureterolithotomy). Chronically obstructed kidneys secondary to ureteric stones can be removed laparoscopically.

Open surgery

Rarely used except again for the reasons above or where laparoscopic skill is unavailable and occasionally to remove a non-functioning kidney.

Metabolic evaluation of stone formers

All patients who present with urinary tract stone disease should have a minimum metabolic assessment to identify any correctable factors, given the high likelihood of further stone episodes in this population. Patients can be stratified into low- and high-risk groups for further stone formation and based on this have a tailored metabolic evaluation (Box 12.5). It is important to adequately evaluate young recurrent stone formers especially those with a family history to rule out abnormal calcium metabolism and less commonly cystinuria. Those patients that have identified metabolic abnormalities can have directed advice and treatment to minimise the risk of further stone episodes. The mainstay of advice is to maintain a high fluid intake to ensure that the urine remains dilute so that the constituents that precipitate into stones are less likely to do so. There is clear evidence that this strategy yields results by decreasing recurrent stone formation.

Box 12.5 **Recommended stone evaluation**

Low-risk patient

First-time stone former: serum creatinine, calcium, urate, urine cystine, urinary pH and stone analysis

High-risk patient

Paediatric stones, recurrent stones, positive family history, history of gout, recurrent UTIs, cystine stones, black patients, chronic malabsorption states and inflammatory bowel disease (raises urinary oxalate levels), hyperparathyroidism, nephrocalcinosis: the above basic metabolic evaluation and two 24-hour collections looking at calcium, magnesium, citrate and oxalate levels and urate, sodium and postassium levels. Total urine volume is measured and is a marker of oral intake.

1% of first time stone presenters have primary hyperparathyroidism on basic metabolic screening.

Cystinuria – an autosomal recessive disorder of cystine transport, preventing its absorption from the proximal renal tubule. High urinary levels result in the precipitation of hard cystine stones.

Further reading

Wein AJ, Kavoussi LR, Novick AC, Partin AW and Peters CA. *Campbell-Walsh Urology*. Ninth Edition. Philadelphia, Saunders (Elsevier), 2007.

Reynard J, Brewster S and Biers S. *Oxford Handbook of Urology*. Oxford, Oxford University Press, 2006.

Türk C, Knoll T, Petrik A et al. *Guidelines on Urolithiasis*. Arnhem, The Netherlands,European Association of Urology, 2010. www.uroweb.org.

CHAPTER 13

The Role of Laparoscopy in Urology

Richard Johnston and Nimish Shah

OVERVIEW

- Laparoscopic surgery leads to shorter hospital stays and faster recovery
- Nearly any open operation can be performed laparoscopically
- Laparoscopic surgery causes certain unique physiologic considerations
- Laparoscopic surgery is still a developing field with many exciting developments

---

History

Because of the retroperitoneal and deep pelvic location of urological organs, open surgery has traditionally required large and morbid incisions.

By the 1950s laparoscopy was limited to diagnostic procedures practised by gastroenterologists. It was a German gynaecologist, Semm, who performed the first laparoscopic appendicectomy in 1983. In 1986 a general surgeon performed the first laparoscopic cholecystectomy.

In 1990, after extensive laboratory trials, the first laparoscopic nephrectomy was performed in the USA. Almost immediately the first laparoscopic varicocelectomy was reported. In 1995 Kavoussi performed the first donor nephrectomy. At many centres, laparoscopic donor nephrectomy is now the standard of care.

The next 20 years saw a paradigm shift in the surgical practise of urology. Minimally invasive surgery initially polarised surgeons into open or laparoscopic camps. It is now clear that the good practice of each has improved the other immensely (see Table 13.1).

Physiological considerations

Carbon dioxide (CO_2) is the gas most commonly used for laparoscopy. It has many advantageous properties – it is colourless, non-combustible and cheap. CO_2 is quickly absorbed and easily diffuses into body tissues (which lessens the chance of a gas

Table 13.1 History of laparoscopic milestones in the UK.

1992	First laparoscopic nephrectomy
1994	First laparoscopic pyeloplasty
2000	First laparoscopic radical prostatectomy

embolus) but may lead to complications including hypercapnia, hypercarbia and associated cardiac arrhythmias.

Pressure effects on organ systems

- Pulmonary – Superior displacement of diaphragm may decrease functional lung capacity and cause higher airway pressure
- Cardiac – Increased resistance to flow in abdominal vasculature may reduce venous return, increasing cardiac work and subsequently blood pressure. Reduced venous return can cause venous pooling in the legs leading to increased deep vein thrombosis (DVT)/pulmonary embolism (PE) risk
- Renal – Pressure effect on renal arteries leads to decreased blood flow, which reduces glomerular filtration rate (GFR) and also causes increased sodium retention. Release of antidiuretic hormone causes water reabsorption. These effects decrease urine output.

Other effects

- GI – Reduced bowel handling results in less sympathetic system activation, with lower rate of ileus. Patient returns to a normal diet faster than after an open operation.
- Immune system – Less intra-operative dissection and manipulation, and lower postoperative pain, leads to faster return of cytokine levels to normal. Although no direct evidence exists, many proponents of laparoscopic surgery believe this leads to improved oncological outcomes.

See Tables 13.2 and 13.3.

Laparoscopic total or partial radical nephrectomy

Total nephrectomy

Laparoscopic treatment of early stage (T1–2) renal tumours should be considered the gold standard. Compared to an open approach, the procedure offers decreased blood loss, less postoperative pain

Table 13.2 Limitations of laparoscopic surgery.

Absolute contraindications	Relative contraindications
Uncorrectable coagulopathy	Morbid obesity
Abdominal wall infection	Extensive prior abdominal surgery
Massive haemoperitoneum (or haemoretroperitoneum)	Hepatomegaly, splenomegaly or intestinal obstruction
Generalised peritonitis	Benign ascites
Suspected malignant ascites	Pregnancy
Intestinal obstruction	Trauma/diaphragmatic hernia (risk of gas entering mediastinum or pleura)
Acute glaucoma	
Raised intracranial pressure	Chronic obstructive pulmonary disease

Table 13.3 Urological procedures that can be performed laparoscopically.

Malignant conditions	Benign conditions
Adrenal tumours	Benign kidney surgery
Nephrectomy – radical or partial	Total nephrectomy
Nephroureterectomy (for transitional cell cancer)	Partial nephrectomy/cyst excision
Cystectomy – radical or partial	Pyeloplasty
Prostatectomy	Stone surgery
Retroperitoneal lymph nodes dissection (RPLND – for testicular cancer)	Donor nephrectomy
	Paediatric surgery
	Undescended testis
	Antireflux surgery
	Female incontinence surgery (e.g. abdominal colposacropexy)
	Varicocele repair

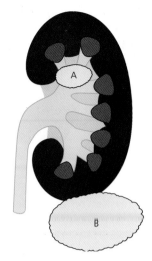

Figure 13.2 A: Small central tumour requiring radical nephrectomy. B: Large exophytic lesion treatable by partial nephrectomy.

and faster recovery. As skills and equipment have improved, more difficult cases (e.g. tumours with renal vein tumour thrombus) have been performed laparoscopically. Oncological equivalence between laparoscopic and open approach has been proven for T1–2 tumours and early evidence supports the continued push to deal with larger tumours and more complex cases (see Figures 13.1 and 13.2).

Partial nephrectomy

Increased use of abdominal imaging has led to more frequent diagnosis of small renal masses. These small lesions are often exophytic; 25% are benign, 25% indolent, and 50% non-indolent. The benefits of a partial nephrectomy include retaining nephrons that would otherwise have been removed. However, the increased laparoscopic skill required, longer warm ischaemia, and potentially additional kidney damage from the pneumoperitoneal pressure often make open partial nephrectomy the preferred technique. Initially laparoscopic partial nephrectomy was only performed for lesions less than 2 cm, although the location of the lesion is now the determining factor (see Figure 13.3).

Laparoscopic donor nephrectomy

Over the past 50 years, since cadaveric nephrectomy has become available, there has been an increasing gap between supply and demand for donors. Living donor nephrectomy (altruistic nephrectomy) has been developed as a method to address this shortfall. Laparoscopic living donor nephrectomy (LLDN) removes some of the disincentives inherent to donation by reducing postoperative pain, shortening hospital stay and improving the cosmetic outcome to the donor.

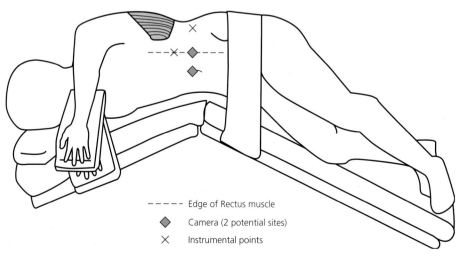

- - - - - Edge of Rectus muscle
◆ Camera (2 potential sites)
✕ Instrumental points

Figure 13.1 Positioning for left kidney laparoscopic surgery.

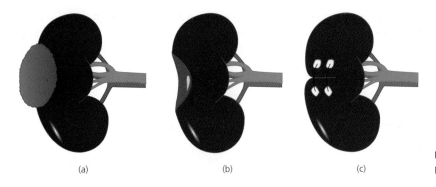

(a)   (b)   (c)

Figure 13.3 Steps required in reconstructing kidney after partial nephrectomy.

LLDN can be performed on either side, transperitoneally or retroperitoneally. The most common approach is left transperitoneal (see Figure 13.4). Live donor transplantation is associated with better short- and long-term renal function for the recipient compared to cadaveric transplantation. Risk factors potentially affecting graft function after LLDN have been shown to be the same as those in open surgery. Increased donor/recipient age, suboptimal immunological match and longer ischaemia time are all associated with impaired renal function/rejection. Compared to open surgery there is a longer ischaemic time with LLDN of approximately three minutes which may lead to reduced graft function. However, no early or late complications have been proven to be due to this.

The contraindications to kidney donation are similar for both open and laparoscopic procedures and focus on maintaining acceptable long-term renal function in the donor. Most donors eligible for an open surgical procedure may undergo a laparoscopic operation instead. Previous contraindications to LLDN, such as right donor kidney, multiple vessels, anomalous vasculature and obesity have been overcome with increasing experience and better equipment.

Complications for the donor include a risk of conversion to open (reported rate of 0–13%). There is concern about the long-term function of the donor's remaining kidney. The relative short duration of follow-up means this question will not be fully answered for another 20 to 30 years.

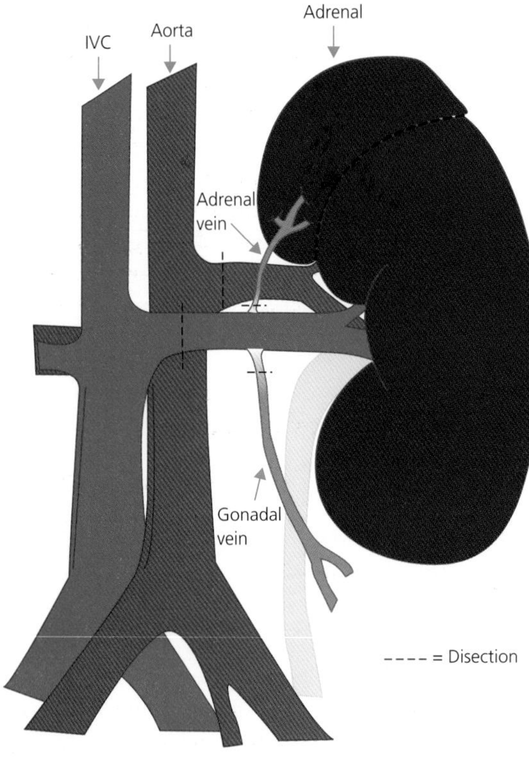

Cysts

Renal cysts are fluid-filled lesions in the kidney. Most are benign simple cysts that need no monitoring or treatment. Cysts can be classified by the Bosniak classification system (based on CT criteria). Those graded III and IV should be removed as a partial or total radical nephrectomy due to a higher risk of malignancy. Congenital cystic disease such as polycystic kidney seldom need surgical management (see Box 13.1)

Box 13.1 Bosniak Grading Scale

Grade I:
   Simple cyst with thin wall. No enhancement. Water density.
Grade II:
   Cyst with a few thin septa or may contain fine calcifications. No enhancement. Hyperdense cysts also in this group.
Grade IIF: (also called grade II follow-up)
   Same as grade II but septa in the cyst may be thick and nodular. There is no enhancement. Any grade II cyst larger than 3 cm.
Grade III:
   Indeterminate cystic masses with thickened irregular septa with enhancement
Grade IV:
   Malignant cystic masses with all the characteristics of category III lesions but also with enhancing soft tissue components independent but adjacent to the septa.

Bosniak I and II cysts occasionally will need treatment, either because they have become so large as to be symptomatic, or the cyst is overlying the exact tract a percutaneous access would take. In this situation cyst decortication is required prior to definitive stone treatment. Percutaneous access to a potentially infected stone through a cyst may cause a chronic cystic infection postoperatively therefore a laparoscopic approach to the kidney is used. The cyst is

IVC   Aorta   Adrenal

Adrenal vein

Gonadal vein

- - - - = Dissection

Figure 13.4 Dissection required for a donor nephrectomy.

opened and marsupialised – meaning the opening is permanently sutured open. A complication of this surgery is re-accumulation of the cyst.

Prostate cancer

Laparoscopic radical prostatectomy aims to replicate open radical retropubic prostatectomy whilst reducing the morbidity associated with surgery. Since its introduction, laparoscopic radical prostatectomy has undergone numerous modifications, most notably a robotic-assisted platform (Da Vinci).

Oncologic survival data for prostate cancer requires a long period of follow-up of at least 20 years. Most laparoscopic series have only 5–15 years follow-up data and so no definitive comparisons can be made. All existing data suggest that robotic, laparoscopic and open prostatectomy are similar in terms of survival.

The advantage of the laparoscopic approach is magnification of the operative field, which allows for a superior dissection, leading to better preservation of the nerves that supply erections, and improved postoperative continence. Roughly 70% of men undergoing bilateral nerve-sparing surgery are able to engage in sexual intercourse at 12–18 months. The results from unilateral nerve-sparing are worse with about 50% success. No matter how well the operation is performed there is always some degree of minor nerve damage and men with difficulty getting erection preoperatively have much worse postoperative results.

Continence result reporting varies greatly, depending on the exact definition used. Most series report slightly better outcomes with laparoscopic approach compared to open surgery.

Laparoscopic radical and partial cystectomy

Laparoscopic radical cystectomy is a technically advanced laparoscopic procedure that requires highly developed laparoscopic skills. It is a long procedure and requires an expert team to get good results.

Open or laparoscopic cystectomy has a significant complication rate of 25–50%, including 2–5% mortality.

Although technically feasible, laparoscopic bladder surgery has significant disadvantages and is performed in only a few expert centres worldwide.

Laparoscopic adrenalectomy

Laparoscopic adrenalectomy has become increasingly popular and is now considered to be the standard technique for removal of adrenal lesions. Adrenal lesions may be functional (e.g. aldosterone secreting and phaeochromocytoma), a primary adrenal malignancy or metastatic. All of these can be removed laparoscopically.

Laparoscopic management for stone disease of urinary tract

Historically stones were managed with open surgical procedures. The invention of shock wave lithotripsy (SWL), endoscopic equipment and minimally invasive procedures such as percutaneous nephrolithotomy (PCNL) has made these operations largely redundant. Laparoscopic stone management should be utilised in cases where SWL, PCNL and ureteroscopy have failed or are deemed unsuitable.

The most common indication for laparoscopic stone surgery is during pyeloplasty repair. Other indications are often arbitrary and depend on the available expertise and equipment. Indications include failed PCNL, ectopic (pelvic) kidneys and caliceal diverticula stones or large (>15 mm upper ureteric) stones.

Laparoscopic pyeloplasty

Uretero-pelvic junction obstruction (UPJ-O) is obstruction of urine moving from the renal pelvis to the upper ureter. The aetiology is complex and two main theories exist: an aberrant renal artery causing obstruction or congenital muscle abnormality preventing normal peristalsis. The outcome is a dilated renal collecting system (hydronephrosis). Untreated, this may cause progressive renal damage and eventual total loss of kidney function.

Prenatal ultrasonography identifies most cases of UPJ-O. Those not screened, or who develop UPJ-O later in life, may present with symptoms of episodic flank or abdominal pain, a palpable flank mass or recurrent UTIs.

Treatment of UPJ-O is not always required. Indications for surgery include progressive loss of renal function, the development of calculi or infection and persistent pain. Treatment techniques, such as percutaneous endopyelotomy, retrograde ureteroscopic endopyelotomy and balloon dilatation exist to treat UPJ-O. However, they have all been shown to have a lower success rates than pyeloplasty. They may still be considered for certain cases. Poor renal function of the affected kidney (<15%) is an indication for nephrectomy rather than pyeloplasty. Failed previous UPJ-O treatment can prove technically challenging but is not a contraindication to laparoscopic pyeloplasty (see Figure 13.5).

There is no randomised comparison between open and laparoscopic pyeloplasty but non-randomised data suggest similar results. Complications include bleeding (5%), urinary leakage (10%) and recurrence (2–15%). The conversion rate to open surgery is 0–4%.

Other laparoscopic procedures

Most open reconstructive and continence procedures have been reported laparoscopically. Laparoscopic repair of testicular vein varicocele is well described but super-selective radiological embolisation is considered the standard of care in the UK.

Future advances

The aim of minimally invasive laparoscopic surgery is shorter hospital stay and convalescence, less pain and better cosmetic results. Current refinements include the use of non-linear instruments

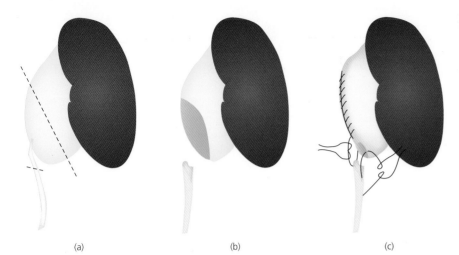

(a)   (b)   (c)   **Figure 13.5** Steps in pyeloplasty repair.

through a single umbilical incision called laparoscopic endoscopic single site surgery (LESS). Currently LESS costs more, takes longer and requires more skill, with no significant improvement in measured outcomes. Other techniques under development include magnetic retractors, non-rigid tools, entering the peritoneum via the stomach, and removing the specimen via the vagina or other orifice.

Further reading

Smith's General Urology, 17th edition, Chapter 9, E. Tanagho and J. McAninch (eds). McGraw-Hill, 2008.

Textbook of Laparoscopic Urology, 1st edition. I Gill (ed.). Informa Healthcare, 2006.

Text book of Practical Laparoscopic Surgery, 2nd edition, R. Mishra (ed.). McGraw-Hill, 2009.

CHAPTER 14

Paediatric Urology

Peter Cuckow

OVERVIEW

- Antenatal hydronephrosis is found on 1% of fetal scans during pregnancy but is transient in most cases
- Urinary tract infection and underlying abnormalities are found in 40% of children with severe UTI
- A tight foreskin is common in young boys but only 1% will require circumcision
- Persistent bedwetting beyond the age of 4 is common and rarely represents a long-term problem
- Cancer in children is rare, the commonest being Wilms' tumour

Introduction

The urological issues in childhood are congenital, acquired or developmental in origin. Presentation may be during a pregnancy screening ultrasound, following routine medical examinations, or later with urinary tract infection, incontinence or symptoms. Knowledge of embryology and development is important to understand both common and rare conditions. Many problems are treated conservatively. Where surgery is required the priorities are preserving renal function, preventing symptoms, and facilitating normal development and long-term function.

Antenatal hydronephrosis

Routine ultrasound is performed twice during pregnancy – an initial dating scan and an anomaly scan between 16 and 20 weeks. Antenatal hydronephrosis (AHN) is the most frequent abnormal finding in up to 1% of fetuses. Abnormal scans enable follow-up and counselling during pregnancy. Although most AHN is transient there is a correlation between its severity and the level of postnatal problems. The ultrasound features give clues as to the underlying pathology: dilatation limited to the renal pelvis is probably due to pelvi-ureteric junction obstruction (PUJ), whereas dilatation involving the pelvis and ureter either to vesico-ureteric

junction obstruction (VUJO) or vesico-ureteric reflux (VUR). If the dilatation is bilateral, bladder outlet obstruction is possible, particularly with a thick walled or non-cycling bladder. In boys this usually occurs because of posterior urethral valves (PUV). Multicystic dysplastic kidney (MCDK), duplex renal collecting systems and ureteroceles have characteristic appearances and reduced or absent liquor can indicate poor urine output and renal insufficiency.

Termination of pregnancy or relief of infravesical obstruction by vesico-amniotic shunting can be offered in severe cases. The latter option is currently unproven but is the subject of clinical studies. At birth prophylactic trimethoprim is started (at a dose of 2 mg/kg weight, daily) and an ultrasound repeated on day 5. With ureteric dilatation, duplex kidneys or bilateral hydronephrosis, a micturating cystogram (MCUG) is performed to document VUR and bladder outlet obstruction. Ultrasound is repeated after 6 weeks in all cases, and again at 3 months if the 6-week scan is still abnormal. Functional imaging is left until 3 months of age to allow for renal maturation – dynamic MAG3 scanning is preferred for patients with obstruction and DMSA scan for VUR. The final diagnoses are summarised in Table 14.1.

Pelvi-ureteric junction obstruction (PUJ)

PUJ obstruction is the commonest cause of PUJ obstruction. Long term studies have shown that most cases of PUJ obstruction resolve spontaneously and the studies have also identified kidneys which are at risk of developing problems The indications to operate are an antero-posterior renal pelvic diameter greater than 30 mm, a differential function below 40%, and calyceal or severe intra-renal dilatation or deterioration on follow-up. Anderson-Hynes dismembered pyeloplasty is the operation of choice, excising the stenotic PUJ and creating a wide anastomosis (see Figure 13.5, Chapter 13).

Table 14.1 Percentages of diagnoses.

PUJ obstruction	38%
Reflux	21%
VUJ obstruction	11%
PUV	10%
Duplex systems	8%
Cystic dysplastic kidney	12%

ABC of Urology, Third Edition.
Edited by Chris Dawson and Janine M. Nethercliffe.
© 2012 John Wiley & Sons, Ltd. Published 2012 by John Wiley & Sons, Ltd.

Dilatation less than 15 mm never deteriorates on follow-up and the patient may be discharged after initial reassuring scans, but this leaves a large number of patients with intermediate dilatation requiring regular follow-up. Deterioration rarely occurs after 4 years of age. In older children PUJ presents with intermittent loin pain, often caused by lower pole vessels compressing the ureter below the pelvis. In these cases (often treated laparoscopically) the anastomosis is made anterior to the vessels.

Vesico-ureteric reflux (VUR)

A deficient valve at the vesico-ureteric junction (VUJ) permits retrograde flow of urine to the kidney. A common end point of the investigation of antenatal hydronephrosis, reflux is usually treated conservatively with prophylactic antibiotics. Maturation of the VUJ gives a high rate of spontaneous resolution during the first five years of life, although this is rare in kidneys with severe dilatation and abnormal function at diagnosis. It is important to rule out posterior urethral valves in boys with reflux, by seeing the whole urethra on MCUG.

A refluxing VUJ is often associated with abnormal kidney development and reduced function on imaging, even without a history of urinary tract infection. Patients with reflux are at risk of secondary renal damage through ascending infection and intra-renal reflux of infected urine. This produces a characteristic pattern of renal scarring at the poles, occurring maximally during the first infective episode but mitigated by prompt antibiotic treatment.

Prophylactic antibiotics are given until after potty training, with surgery indicated for breakthrough infection, non-compliance, deterioration in dilatation or function on follow-up imaging, and non-resolution of the reflux.

First-line surgery is endoscopic injection of an inert paste below the refluxing orifice. Open surgery is reserved for more severe cases, where injection is not possible, or following failed injection treatment. The distress of MCUG and catheterisation is avoided in older children by using MAG3 indirect cystography instead. VUR and its renal consequences remain a major cause of end stage renal failure in children.

Posterior urethral valves

Posterior urethral valves cause hydro-ureteronephrosis and secondary VUR in boys and the valves are easily missed on an inadequate MCUG. Renal and bladder abnormalities are increased with earlier and more severe antenatal dilatation and bad cases may present at birth with renal failure and respiratory distress (due to pulmonary hypoplasia). The initial management is catheter drainage to optimise native renal function before endoscopic valve ablation. Advances in neonatal care and renal failure management have improved survival until transplant can be performed in severe cases. Diversion by vesicostomy or ureterostomy is rarely indicated although bladder reconstruction has an important role to create a safe reservoir to optimise poorly functioning kidneys or for the transplant.

VUJ obstruction

Characterised by a visible dilated ureter to the level of the bladder and often lesser renal dilatation, VUJ obstruction (otherwise

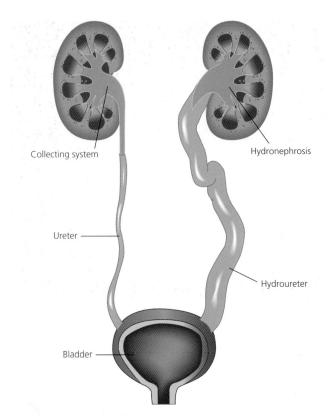

Figure 14.1 Obstruction of the vesico-ureteric junction.

known as megaureter or hydro-ureteronephrosis) is more benign than PUJ (Figure 14.1). With prophylactic antibiotics the dilatation my resolve spontaneously, although some patients with diminished renal function or breakthrough infection will come to surgery in early life. Early intervention may be a simple drainage procedure such as ipsilateral ureterostomy or open JJ stent insertion. This delays bladder surgery (tapered ureteric reimplantation), which may harm early bladder development but is usually very successful.

Urinary tract duplication

Duplicated collecting systems occur in 1 in 100 girls and 1 in 200 boys. In severe cases both functional imaging and cystography are needed to determine renal function, ureteric and bladder anatomy (Figure 14.2). Most commonly the ureters join before the bladder (partial duplication) and associated problems are rare. In complete duplication lower ureters share a common blood supply and cross so the upper pole orifice is below and medial to the lower pole orifice on the trigone (the Meyer-Weigert law) (Figure 14.3). The abnormally placed ureteric orifice is related to the degree of dysplasia of the renal unit. Lower poles are prone to reflux, which less often resolves spontaneously but may be treated with endoscopic injection. Lower pole nephro-ureterectomy is indicated for poor function and laparoscopy enables low ureteric division, reducing stump complications. Some upper pole ureters end in a ureterocele and this is usually associated with negligible polar function for which upper pole heminephrectomy is often indicated. Ureteroceles may obstruct the bladder outlet and threaten all renal moieties so endoscopic puncture is used for

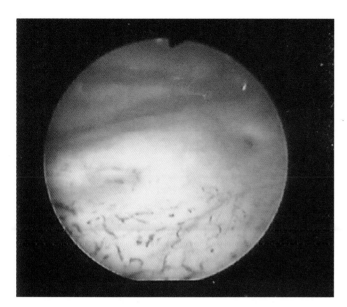

Figure 14.2 Cystoscopic views of duplex left ureteric orifices.

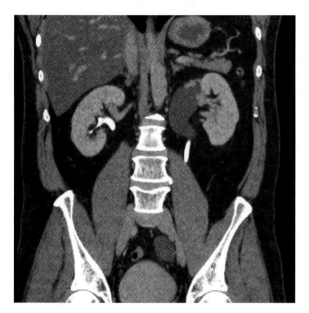

Figure 14.3 Duplication of the ureters.

early decompression. This can create reflux and some patients will require open bladder surgery in addition to hemi-nephrectomy to excise the ureterocele, repair the trigone and reimplant the lower pole ureter

Multicystic dysplastic kidney

MCDK is the usual cause of unilateral renal agenesis. These cystic kidneys have no function and commonly regress and become invisible on ultrasound either during pregnancy or the first two years. With a normal contralateral kidney the outcome is usually good and surgery (usually laparoscopic nephrectomy) is indicated for huge kidneys over 6 cm that never regress and those that persist beyond 2 years. Theoretical long-term issues of hypertension and tumour transformation are probably extremely rare.

Table 14.2 Anomalies associated with UTI.

VUR	29% (VUR plus scarring 14.5%)
PUJ/VUJ anomalies	4.5%
Duplication anomalies	4.5%
Other	2%

Urinary tract infection (UTI)

UTI occurs in 2% of boys and 8% of girls. Most boys present below 1 year of age, but for girls presentation is usually later, around school age. Before antenatal diagnosis, UTI was a common presentation of urinary tract anomalies. Investigation of children with severe UTI reveals an abnormality in 40% (see Table 14.2).

Early and more severe UTIs are most commonly associated with anomalies and in 2007 the National Institute for Health and Clinical Excellence (NICE) published guidelines to avoid unnecessary invasive tests. MCUG and functional studies should be reserved for children under 1 year of age, severe symptoms, recurrent UTI and patients whose initial ultrasound shows an abnormality. Although urine dipsticks enable early diagnosis, a laboratory culture should be performed to secure the diagnosis and confirm the correct antibiotic. Gut organisms predominate and the commonest is *E. coli*.

Later presenting urinary tract infection is often associated with dysfunctional elimination, where children fail to develop regular voiding or bowel habits and may be both wet and constipated. Rigorous behavioural management is the first priority to avoid recurrent and long-term problems and the addition of prophylactic antibiotics and aperients in some cases. Probiotics and vitamin C are useful adjuncts to help prevent infection.

Abnormalities of the genitalia

The foreskin

Normal foreskin development is poorly understood. Non-retraction and adhesions between glans and inner prepuce are usual during the early years. Only 1% of boys require circumcision for scarring that prevents retraction in older boys (balanitis xerotica et obliterans). Whilst balanitis (inflammation of the glans and prepuce of uncertain aetiology) and ballooning may cause distress during childhood, reassurance should be the principal approach, as these common issues resolve without long-term implications. Circumcision causes significant complications in some patients and meatal stenosis requiring a formal meatoplasty is needed in 2–5% of cases.

Testes

Testicular descent occurs before three months in a hormonally led sequence, so undescended testis (UDT) is more common in prematurity and reduces to an incidence of 1% by 6 months. Neonatal and GP examinations prompt specialist referral, but careful examination often finds normal mobile testes. Those manipulated comfortably into the scrotum are retractile and need no surgery. Open orchidopexy is effective for true UDT, between 6 and 18 months.

Ten per cent of UDTs are impalpable. The investigation of choice is laparoscopy to find an intra-abdominal testis or confirm its absence or atrophy (the latter possibly due to torsion). During the same procedure a first-stage orchidopexy is performed for intra-abdominal testis, or orchidectomy for severe abnormality. If the testis is absent the normal side is fixed, to reduce the risk of later torsion. Staged orchidopexy is completed 6 months later with a success rate of 80%.

Statistically, fertility is reduced and testis cancer increased 5–10-fold in UDT. In individual cases the risk is probably proportional to the severity of testicular abnormality.

As testes descend there is an extension of the peritoneal cavity along the cord to the scrotum, called the processus vaginalis, which usually closes in early life. A wide persistent processus can allow herniation of abdominal contents and needs urgent surgery to prevent incarceration or strangulation. A narrow communication allowing fluid to collect around the testis is the origin of a childhood (communicating) hydrocele. Seen commonly in the neonatal period these mostly resolve during the first year of life. Surgery (herniotomy) should be reserved for persistence or massive size.

Acute scrotal pain and swelling in childhood are most commonly caused by idiopathic scrotal oedema or torsion of the testicular appendage. Epididymo-orchitis is relatively rare. Torsion of the testis itself is most common around puberty. Although there are specific features to differentiate between these, clinical uncertainty and the need to be safe often lead to diagnostic exploration, and fixation of both testes where torsion is confirmed.

Hypospadias

An abnormal ventral development of the penis, hypospadias is characterised by a dorsal hooded foreskin, a proximally placed urethral opening and a degree of ventral curvature (chordee) and occurs in 1 in 300 males. Severe types with ambiguous genitalia at birth and particularly those with asymmetric gonads need to be investigated as for disorders of sexual differentiation (DSD, below). In most cases (80%) the meatus is in the distal penis, the curvature is caused by skin-tethering, and a single stage procedure at around 1 year of age has good results. In the remainder a more proximal urinary meatus is associated with significant chordee that needs correction in two stages, 6 months apart. The first stage straightens the corpora, uses the excess skin to graft the ventral penile shaft, and split the glans penis to create a wide urethral plate. This can then be easily closed in layers at the second stage. Although excellent results are reported, hypospadias repair is still associated with significant complications that include meatal stenosis, urethral stricture, urethral fistula and complete breakdown.

Disorders of sexual differentiation (DSD)

The early embryonic genitalia are identical and the default pathway is female development. In males the testis-determining gene on the Y chromosome (SRY) directs gonad development into testes. Müllerian inhibiting substance (MIS) is produced by Sertoli cells and stops uterine, fallopian tube and proximal vaginal development. Testosterone from Leydig cells acts via androgen receptors to form the male penis, urethra and vasal system. DSD (previously known as intersex conditions) result from a defect in this pathway and

present at birth with ambiguous genitalia. It is an urgent matter to resolve the sex of rearing of these babies and management should be by a multi-disciplinary team. Clinical examination, biochemical investigation of blood and urine, karyotype examination, and pelvic ultrasound are the main early investigations. Endocrine stimulation tests and diagnostic laparoscopy are selectively used.

Incontinence

Potty training occurs in most children around two and a half years of age and night-time dryness follows over the next year. Delays in this process to 4 years of age are not necessarily abnormal. Persistent isolated nocturnal enuresis is common, investigations are usually normal, and the problem invariably resolves spontaneously during childhood. Desmopressin, bed alarms and anti-cholinergics may be used but may fail if the children themselves are not motivated.

Daytime wetting is most commonly associated with dysfunctional voiding but may also have an underlying organic cause. Evaluation by careful history and genital examination, augmented by frequency volume charts, urine flow rates and urinary tract ultrasound provide a thorough assessment. Invasive video-urodynamics, using suprapubic lines, is used selectively in severe cases. Functional incontinence is managed by bladder re-training with prophylactic antibiotics, anticholinergics and aperients as required. The rarer organic causes of daytime wetting include major urinary tract anomalies, neuropathic bladder, ectopic ureter in girls and posterior urethral valves in boys.

Neuropathic bladder

This is associated with spina bifida, sacral agenesis, ano-rectal anomalies, spinal tumours, or rare infections such as transverse myelitis. In these patients bladder dysfunction is suspected. Sometimes abnormal video-urodynamics prompts a diagnostic spinal MRI. There is a range of abnormality dependent on bladder capacity and sphincter and detrusor function. Urodynamic assessment guides treatment; overactive bladder can be mitigated with anticholinergic therapy, and poor emptying by clean intermittent catheterisation – these are mainstays of conservative management. In patients with small capacity or high-pressure bladders augmentation with ileum may be necessary either for persistent incontinence, or more acutely when upper tracts are compromised. A catheterisable appendix (Mitrofanoff) channel provides effective emptying. Sphincter weakness is rarely managed by artificial sphincter in children and a synchronous bladder neck procedure is preferred. Botox injections to the detrusor are still being evaluated.

Bladder exstrophy and epispadias

Primary bladder exstrophy is a rare abnormality of the abdominal wall and pelvis, occurring in 1 in 30 000 births. The pelvic ring is open and the rectus muscles are apart below the umbilicus, with an open bladder plate filling the space in the midline. The penis is open dorsally in continuity with the bladder plate. Reconstruction is complex and limited to two UK centres.

Primary epispadias is a similar but rarer condition where the urethra is variably deficient on its dorsal aspect. In all girls and many boys the bladder neck is involved and they are incontinent. Reconstruction has to address both the genital and continence issues. Severe dorsal curvature is a major feature of the penile problem. Many patients end up with a cystoplasty and Mitrofanoff.

Cancer

Wilms' tumour of the kidney (WT)

This is the commonest paediatric urological malignancy of childhood with 8 cases per million population annually. Presentation is between 1 and 5 years of age with an abdominal mass and occasionally abdominal pain and hypertension. Wilms' tumour is associated with a number of syndromes.

Imaging is by ultrasound, CT or MRI to confirm the diagnosis, detect tumour spread, and establish operability. The differential diagnoses include mesoblastic nephroma (a benign tumour presenting before 6 months) and neuroblastoma outside the kidney (characterised by raised urinary substances secreted from the tumour).

The tumour stage at surgery and its histological type determine the extent of chemotherapy and radiotherapy. Survival greater than 85% at 5 years is achieved in most patients. Bilateral cases (accounting for 10% of Wilms' tumours) have a survival rate of over 70% but require more conservative partial nephrectomies to preserve renal function.

Rhabdomyosarcoma (RMS)

Genito-urinary RMS occurs below the age of 10 in 1 per million population per year and presents with urinary dysfunction, haematuria, pelvic/abdominal mass or a visible perineal growth. Imaging and biopsy then chemotherapy is followed by an excision of residual tumour. Radiotherapy has an important role. Tumour clearance with preservation of bladder function and continence can be achieved, although radical excision and urinary diversion is needed in severe or relapsing cases. Overall survival is over 60%.

Further reading

Pediatric Urology. Gearhart JP, Rink RC and Mouriquand PDE (eds). WB Saunders, 2001.

NICE Guidelines on the Investigation of Urinary Tract Infection in Children. www.nice.org.uk

Cuckow PC, Nyirady P and Winyard PJD. Normal and abnormal development of the urogenital tract. *Prenat Diag* 2001; 21: 908–16.

Woodward M and Frank D. Postnatal management of antenatal hydronephrosis. *BJU International* 2002; 89: 149–56.

Brain CE, Creighton SM, Mushtaq I et al Holistic management of DSD. *Best Pract Res Clin Endocrinol Metab* 2010; 24(2): 335–54.

Hutson JM, Balic A, Nation T and Southwell B. Cryptorchidism. *Seminars in Ped Surg* 2010; 19: 215–24.

Ahmed HU, Arya M, Tsiouris A et al. An update on the management of Wilms' tumour. *Eur J Surg Oncol* 2007; 33: 824–31.

Baskin LS and Ebbers MB. Hypospadias: anatomy, etiology and technique. *J Ped Surg* 2006; 41: 463–72.

CHAPTER 15

Urological Trauma

Tamsin Greenwell

OVERVIEW

- Stricture resulting from any anterior urethral injury will require deferred urethroplasty
- The majority of posterior urethral injuries result from road traffic accidents
- Injuries to the bladder are rare following abdominal injury, but blunt trauma is most commonly the cause
- Most ureteric injuries are iatrogenic, occurring after surgery, and may present with obstruction or a with a fistula
- The majority of cases of blunt renal trauma are minor but significant injury may occur in up to 68% of cases of penetrating trauma and 25% of patients with blunt trauma

Urethral trauma

Anterior urethral injury

Anterior urethral injuries may be classified as either partial or complete disruption. The aetiology of these injuries is shown in Box 15.1.

Box 15.1 Aetiology of anterior urethral injuries

- Blunt trauma: fall astride, kick to perineum
- Penetrating trauma: gunshot wound, stab wound
- Sexual trauma: foreign body, penile fracture, constriction band
- Iatrogenic: urethral catheter, endoscopic surgery, penile surgery

---

The history of the injury will suggest the mechanism of the injury. An inability to void is a significant feature. Examination should be performed to look for blood at the urethral meatus and may also show a haematoma or urinoma confined to Buck's or Colles' fascia (Figure 15.1).

One gentle attempt at urethral catheterisation is permitted in these circumstances but if any difficulty is encountered then a

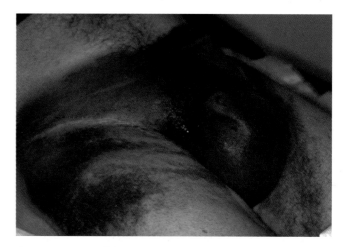

Figure 15.1 Bruising following anterior urethral injury.

suprapubic catheter should be inserted. If a penetrating injury has occurred then immediate debridement is required.

Immediate repair of the injury is indicated if:

- The patient is stable
- There is a penetrating injury
- If debridement is required
- If there is minimal haematoma
- If there is associated fracture of the penis.

If the urethra is extensively damaged then the area should be debrided and the urethra marsupialised.

Definitive management of these injuries is by urethroplasty of any stricture, waiting for a minimum of 3 months.

Posterior urethral injury

The classification of these injuries is shown in Box 15.2.

Box 15.2 Classification of posterior urethral injury

1 Stretched but intact
2 Partial disruption
3 Complete disruption
4 Complex (involving the bladder neck or rectum)

ABC of Urology, Third Edition.
Edited by Chris Dawson and Janine M. Nethercliffe.
© 2012 John Wiley & Sons, Ltd. Published 2012 by John Wiley & Sons, Ltd.

Posterior urethral injuries can occur through different aetiologies, shown in Box 15.3.

Box 15.3 **Aetiology of posterior urethral injury**

- Penetrating trauma: gunshot wound, stab wound
- Pelvic fracture related trauma: road traffic accident, fall from height, industrial accident
- Iatrogenic: transurethral resection of prostate (TURP), other endoscopic surgery, radical prostatectomy

---

Pelvic fracture urethral distraction defect (PFUDD)

Pelvic fracture occurs with an incidence of 20–30 per 100 000.

Pelvic fracture urethral distraction defect occurs in 2–25% of patients suffering pelvic fracture. The mechanism of injury is avulsion of the fixed membranous urethra from the more mobile bulbar urethra by vertical force and/or a bony fragment injury. Ten per cent of PFUDD will occur with an isolated pelvic fracture but 90% are associated with multiple injuries. The majority are related to motor vehicle accidents, but other causes include falls and crush injuries.

As most of these injuries occur along with other serious trauma the initial evaluation will include finding out about the mechanism of injury, trauma resuscitation, and the treatment of associated injuries.

PFUDD should be suspected if there is blood at the urethral meatus, an inability to void urine, a palpable bladder, a high-riding prostate on digital rectal examination (DRE), pelvic fracture with displacement of pubic rami, or butterfly bruising of the perineum consistent with haematoma confined to Colles' fascia.

One gentle attempt at urethral catheterisation is permitted but if there is any difficulty inserting the catheter a suprapubic catheter should be inserted. If the patient is stable then a retrograde urethrogram can be performed (see Figure 15.2).

Once the patient is stable then specialist urological opinion should be sought.

The mean rates for restricture, erectile dysfunction and urinary incontinence for different surgical options are shown in Table 15.1.

Iatrogenic posterior urethral injury

This generally occurs in older men, after either open or endoscopic prostatic surgery. The aims of treatment are to restore the urethral

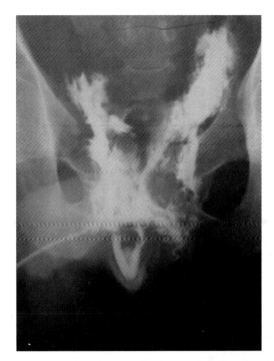

Figure 15.2 Retrograde urethrogram showing complete disruption of the urethra with extravasation of contrast.

continuity with preservation of sphincter function. The initial management is by urethral dilation, followed by clean intermittent self-catheterisation. If this management plan fails, or is unacceptable to the patient, then alternative options include definitive repair accepting the risk of urinary incontinence and the need for artificial urinary sphincter (AUS) or urinary diversion.

Female urethral injuries

Injuries to the female urethra accompany up to 6% of pelvic fractures. Half of these are missed at the time of injury, and all are associated with vaginal injury. A partial tear or mild injury often presents later as urinary incontinence. Box 15.4 shows the classification of these injuries.

Box 15.4 **Classification of female urethral injury**

1 Mild – damage to the nerve supply of urethra only, presenting later as urinary incontinence (25%)
2 Moderate – a longitudinal tear of the urethra, presenting later as urinary incontinence (17%)
3 Severe – urethral avulsion, giving a classic PFUDD picture (58%), at the bladder neck, the proximal urethra or the distal urethra

---

The safest management is insertion of a suprapubic catheter followed by referral for expert delayed repair. Delayed management is usually determined by the degree of urethral injury. Mild and moderate injury usually causes incontinence, and this is managed with a bladder neck AUS. Severe urethral injury, which usually causes an obliterative stricture, requires formal reconstruction. Indications for immediate repair are as for male PFUDD.

Table 15.1 Options for the management of posterior urethral injury and the mean restricture, erectile dysfunction and ureteric dysfunction rates after each.

	Restricture	ED	UI
Primary surgical repair	62%	31%	15%
Delayed primary surgical repair	20%	71%	0%
Primary open realignment	61%	39%	14%
Primary endoscopic realignment	64%	25%	5.6%
Delayed endoscopic repair	82%	36%	5%
Delayed bulbar prostatic anastomosis	17%	14%	9%
ED rates subsequent to fracture alone		33-50%	

ED = erectile dysfunction
UI = urinary iincontinence

Table 15.2 Severity score for bladder trauma.

Grade	Injury type	Description of injury
I	Haematoma	Contusion, intramural haematoma
II	Laceration	Partial thickness
III	Laceration	Extraperitoneal bladder wall laceration <2 cm
IV	Laceration	Intraperitoneal bladder wall laceration >2 cm
V	Laceration	Intra- or extraperitoneal bladder wall laceration extending into the bladder neck or ureteric orifice (trigone)

Bladder trauma

Injuries to the bladder accompany 2% of abdominal injuries. Blunt trauma is the cause in 67–86% and penetrating trauma in 14–33%. Bladder trauma can be extraperitoneal and/or intraperitoneal. Table 15.2 shows the American Association for the Surgery of Trauma (AAST) severity score for bladder trauma.

The initial history should include a description of the mechanism of injury. Examination will often reveal gross haematuria, abdominal tenderness, inability to void, bruising in the suprapubic region and abdominal distension.

Extravasation of urine may cause swelling in the perineum, scrotum, thighs and anterior abdominal wall.

Initial imaging with retrograde cystography has an accuracy of 85–100% and should include bladder filling views (with at least 350 ml of contrast) and post-drainage views. CT cystography is an alternative investigation. Figure 15.3 shows views of extraperitoneal and intraperitoneal rupture.

The management of blunt trauma causing extraperitoneal rupture is urethral catheter drainage for 14–21 days. Operative intervention may be required if there is bladder neck involvement, presence of bone fragments in the bladder wall, or entrapment of the bladder wall by bone.

Penetrating trauma causing extraperitoneal rupture requires operative intervention and repair, as does either blunt or penetrating trauma causing intraperitoneal rupture (risk of peritonitis if left).

A standard, or CT, cystogram is required at 14–21 days post-repair or drainage to assess healing.

Ureteric trauma

Radiotherapy may damage the ureter. The latter is the most radiosensitive abdominal organ as it tolerates only 20–25 Gy, much less than the dose usually administered. Damage is maximal 4–6 cm from the ureteric orifice, at the base of the broad ligament.

The majority of ureteric injuries are, however, iatrogenic occurring after surgery. Fifty-seven per cent of such injuries occur after obstetric procedures, 21% after gynaecological procedures and 7% after ureteroscopy. The incidence of ureteric damage is approximately 0.05–1% after hysterectomy and is greater in abdominal than in laparoscopic hysterectomy.

Ureteric injuries may present as obstruction or with a fistula. An obstruction usually presents within 5 days although a fistula may present later. A fistula almost always co-exists with some degree of obstruction.

The classification of ureteric injuries is shown in Box 15.5.

> **Box 15.5 Classification of ureteric injuries**
>
> **I** Haematoma: contusion or haematoma without devascularisation
> **II** Laceration: <50% transection
> **III** Laceration: >50% transection
> **IV** Laceration: complete transection with <2 cm devascularisation
> **V** Laceration: avulsion with >2 cm devascularisation

The factors affecting successful repair are:

- length (<5 cm high (80%+) success, >5 cm low (40%) success)
- previous radiotherapy reduces successful repair rates (from >80% to 60%)
- time of treatment (immediate repair is associated with the highest success (100%) and late repair the lowest (73%).

Assessment of suspected ureteric injury is normally by IVU or CT urogram. An ultrasound scan may show obstruction to the kidney.

Endoscopic stenting of the damaged segment may be attempted but nephrostomy alone is inadequate. Antegrade stenting of short partial occlusions (e.g. fistulae) is successful in 50–90%. Antegrade and retrograde stenting may be successful in longer strictures where operative intervention is not an immediate option.

Open surgery may be required to repair the damaged ureter; if there is insufficient length for a tension-free anastomosis then the bladder can be bought upwards to compensate ureteric length (Psoas hitch or Boari flap procedures). A Psoas hitch procedure

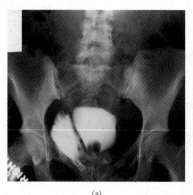
(a)

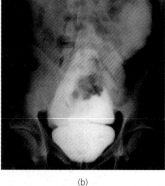
(b)

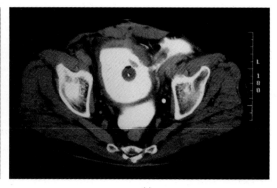
(c)

Figure 15.3 (a) Extraperitoneal rupture; (b) intraperitoneal rupture; (c) CT showing both extra- and intraperitoneal rupture.

may be better as a single technique or in combination as it stabilises the ureteric reimplantation site.

Transureterostomy is sometimes required when pelvic reimplantation proves impossible. Ileal ureteric substitution is rarely performed because of the metabolic complication and the risk of stone formation.

Ureterostomy in situ may be performed in an emergency as a salvage procedure, and nephrectomy may be considered if there is poor renal function in the affected renal unit, or in the elderly or unfit.

Renal trauma

Renal trauma affects 5 per 100 000 of the population and occurs in 1.2–3.25% of trauma patients.

Most cases of renal trauma are blunt injury, resulting from motor vehicle accidents or falls. In the UK, penetrating injuries account for approximately 5% of renal injuries. Pre-existing renal lesions such as hydronephrosis, cysts, tumours and abnormal position are frequently associated with cases of blunt trauma in adults.

The majority of cases of blunt renal trauma are minor, although significant injury occurs in 27–68% of cases of penetrating trauma and in 4–25% of patients with blunt trauma. Associated injuries occur in 20–94%. Box 15.6 shows the classification of renal injury.

During initial evaluation the history should elicit the mechanism of injury and the vital signs should be assessed as well as possible entry and exit wounds, flank bruising or rib fractures.

> **Box 15.6 Classification of renal injury according to the American Association for the Surgery of Trauma (AAST)**
>
> **1** Contusion/haematoma –
> - Normal urological studies, haematuria/subcapsular non-expanding haematoma
>
> **2** Haematoma/laceration –
> - Non-expanding perirenal haematoma confined to retroperitoneum/<1 cm cortex laceration with no urinary extravasation
>
> **3** Laceration
> - 1 cm cortex laceration with no collecting system rupture or urinary extravasation
>
> **4** Laceration/vascular Injury
> - Parenchymal laceration through cortex, medulla and collecting system/main renal artery or vein injury with contained haemorrhage
>
> **5** Laceration/vascular injury
> - Completely shattered kidney/avulsion of hilum which devascularises kidney

Haematuria is present in 80–94% of cases of renal trauma but is absent where there is vascular pedicle injury, and in penetrating injury.

Half of patients with penetrating trauma will have a grade 3 to 5 injury and all require immediate CT and/or surgical exploration (see Box 15.7).

> **Box 15.7 Management of blunt renal trauma**
>
> Blunt trauma in adults (>16 years)
>
> - 12.5% have grade 3–5 injury
> - If gross haematuria, or microhaematuria and systolic BP < 90 mmHg – CT required
> - If microhaematuria and systolic BP >90 mmHg – no imaging required
>
> Blunt trauma in children
>
> - Gross haematuria – CT required
> - Microhaematuria – if >50 rbc/hpf – CT required
> - but if <50 rbc/hpf – no imaging required

Initial imaging should be by contrast CT which is 65–95% accurate. CT may show vascular injury, parenchymal laceration, urinary extravasation or perirenal haematoma, and may also delineate other intra-abdominal injuries – see Figure 15.4.

If emergency surgical exploration is required a one-shot IVU can be performed on-table using a 2 ml/kg bolus of IV contrast and one 10-minute film.

After conservative management a repeat abdominal contrast CT is performed at 36–48 hours for any grade 4–5 renal injury.

The absolute indications for renal exploration are persistent life-threatening haemorrhage, renal pedicle avulsion or an expanding pulsatile haematoma, or uncontained retroperitoneal haematoma.

The relative indications for renal exploration are shown in Box 15.8.

Nephrectomy is required in 13–100% of cases overall. The rate is higher in penetrating injuries, high velocity injuries, or where there is an overall higher severity of injury. If significant arterial injury is present immediate nephrectomy gives the best outcomes. Arterial injury is mandatory where there is bilateral injury, in cases of solitary kidney or cases where simple repair of the artery is possible.

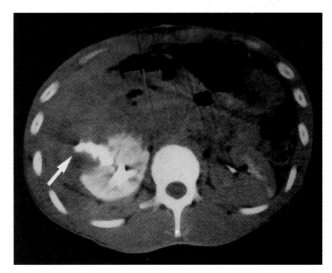

Figure 15.4 Contrast CT showing grade 3 injury.

Follow-up imaging is not required for grade 1 or 2 injuries, or in stable grade 3 injuries with no devitalised segments. Patients with grade 4 or 5 injuries should have a repeat contrast CT scan performed at 26–72 hours and will also require a DMSA renogram.

Secondary haemorrhage occurs in 13–25% of grade 3 or 4 injuries usually due to arterio-venous fistula or pseudo-aneurysm formation. The management of these complications is by embolisation.

Renal ischaemia causes excess renin secretion and may occur due to renal artery thrombosis, renal parenchymal compression by haematoma, or fibrosis. Incidence increases with severity of injury and is on average 5.2% (0.6–33%). Hypertension is a possible sequel to this and follow-up is by periodic BP measurement post-injury. Nephrectomy is the commonest treatment.

Renal failure occurs in 6.4%, and reduced function in 16%. This occurs most commonly after grade 4 and 5 injuries.

Further reading

Consensus Statement on Urethral Trauma. Chapple C, Barbagli G, Jordan G et al. *BJU Int* 2004; 93: 195–202.

Pelvic fracture injuries of the female urethra. Venn SN, Greenwell TJ and Mundy AR. *BJU Int* 1999; 83: 626–30.

Organ injury scaling. III. Chest wall, abdominal, vascular, ureter, bladder and urethra. Moore EE, Cogbill TH, Jurkovich GJ et al. *J Trauma* 1992; 33: 337–9.

Buckley JC and McAninch JW. Revision of Current American Association for the Surgery of Trauma Renal Injury Grading System. *J Trauma* 2011; 70; 35–7.

Ureteral injuries: apropos of 42 cases. Benchekroun A, Lachkar A, Soumana A, Fraihm H, Belahnech Z et al. *Ann Urol (Paris)* 1997; 31: 267–72.

CHAPTER 16

Penile Cancer and Gender Reassignment

Majid Shabbir and Nim Christopher

OVERVIEW

Penile cancer

- A rare condition with ~350 new cases/year in the UK

- Early detection and treatment is essential to ensuring a good outcome. If diagnosis is in doubt, biopsy and early referral to a specialist centre is recommended

- Pooling of resources in specialist centres has substantially improved understanding, techniques and outcomes

- The use of penile preserving surgical techniques, in conjunction with dynamic sentinel lymph node sampling, reduces the impact of treatment and maintains penile form and function with excellent oncological and cosmetic results.

- Close follow-up and early detection of tumour recurrence is essential to ensure favourable long-term outcomes.

Gender reassignment

- Incidence per year in the UK: 1:30 000 for female to male (FTM) and 1:10 000 for male to female (MTF)

- Specialist Gender Identity Clinics are necessary for assessment, diagnosis and initiation of treatment

- Harry Benjamin criteria are used internationally for the whole gender reassignment process

- Genital sex reassignment surgery (SRS) in the UK: 200+/yr for MTF and 50+/yr for FTM patients

- SRS is a complex multi-stage and multi-disciplinary process with best results by dedicated centres

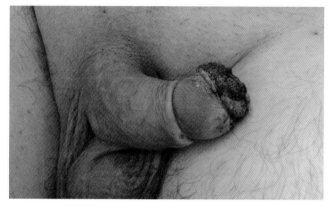

Figure 16.1 Typical exophytic penile cancer lesion.

Penile cancer

Penile cancer is an uncommon malignancy, accounting for <1% of all male cancers in Europe and the US. The key to management is early recognition, which provides the best chance of curative treatment whilst preserving the penis. Matters are not helped by delayed presentation due to embarrassment, fear and stigma associated with genital problems, which can often render a simple treatable lesion into one requiring a more radical surgical approach.

Presentation

Penile cancer can be difficult to detect. Subtle malignant lesions can be difficult to distinguish from benign ones, and the rarity of the condition means that even most urologists only see one new case every two years. More obvious lesions typically grow rapidly, are exophytic, have a warty appearance, and can be very destructive (See Figure 16.1). Subtle cancers, or premalignant lesions, may present with nothing more than a red patch or an innocuous painless ulcer. A high index of suspicion is essential. Any rapidly changing lesion or one which has failed to respond to initial treatment should be biopsied and referred to a specialist centre for an early opinion. Key aspects to note on examination are the size, appearance, colour, number of lesions, their location, what structures they appear to involve and the presence of any mass in the groin.

Risk factors

Penile cancer is more common in men aged 50–70 years, but up to 20% occur in men <40 years. Several risk factors have been associated with penile cancer, and these are highlighted in Box 16.1. Areas of controversy are highlighted in Box 16.2.

Investigations

All patients with suspected penile cancer should have a biopsy to confirm the diagnosis, and give an indication of the tumour type and grade (graded 1–3, well to poorly differentiated).

ABC of Urology, Third Edition.
Edited by Chris Dawson and Janine M. Nethercliffe.
© 2012 John Wiley & Sons, Ltd. Published 2012 by John Wiley & Sons, Ltd.

Approximately 95% are squamous cell carcinomas (SCC), the rest being melanomas, sarcomas or basal cell carcinomas.

Box 16.1 Risk factors for penile cancer

- Presence of foreskin
- Phimosis/poor hygiene
- Sexual history including early age first contact/multiple partners
- HPV infection types 16 & 18
- Chronic inflammation: lichen sclerosus et atrophicus (LSA) (previously known as balanitis xerotica obliterans, BXO)
- Smoking/chewing tobacco
- PUVA (photochemotherapy using ultraviolet light for psoriasis)

Box 16.2 Risk factors – areas of controversy

Human papilloma virus (HPV)
- HPV DNA is found in up to 50% of penile tumours
- HPV vaccinations for penile cancer prevention are effective, but only provide reliable cover for up to 5 years, and need be given before first sexual contact
- As HPV infection is not the only cause of penile cancer, the vaccine gives no guarantee of prevention

Lichen sclerosus et atrophicus (LSA) or balanitis xerotica obliterans (BXO)
- A common cause of phimosis and often seen concurrently with penile cancer
- Contentiously considered to be premalignant
- New tumour developments in LSA very low (<6%), with long latency (mean 17 years)
- Impractical to follow up all. Pragmatically closely follow only those with chronic active disease. Teach remaining, in whom changes regresses after circumcision, self-examination. Biopsy any new or unusual lesions

Circumcision
- Penile cancer is very rare in men circumcised at birth
- Neonatal circumcision reduces relative risk of cancer threefold, but controversial as number needed to treat (NNT) is high due to rarity of cancer
- Circumcision in adult does not prevent penile cancer, but aids treatment/ detection
- Clear benefits of adult circumcision for preventing HPV and HIV infections or preventing/treating chronic inflammatory conditions like LSA associated with penile cancer

---

While an MRI of the penis (performed with an artificial erection) is not essential, it is helpful in identifying the depth of invasion in cases where this is not clinically obvious. A staging CT scan of the chest/abdomen and pelvis is used to assess for metastases, although it has a low sensitivity for detecting lymph node involvement (36%). PET-CT is more accurate, but not widely available and can miss micro-metastases. Surgical staging of regional nodes is often required.

All patients are discussed in specialist multi-disciplinary team (MDT) meetings with the results of these investigations to formulate optimised individual treatment plans.

Treatment

Treatment is in two phases: treating the primary lesion, and tackling the regional lymph nodes. Traditionally, primary lesions were over-treated with radical surgery or radical radiotherapy. A total penectomy was effective oncologically (recurrence rates <1%), but emasculating with serious psychosexual consequences. Although radiotherapy allowed organ preservation the penis never looked or functioned the same again and there was a high risk of local recurrence (~40%) which was difficult to treat.

Pooling of expertise in specialist centres has improved the understanding of penile cancer. The realisation that a margin of only a few millimetres rather than 2 cm was adequate for clearance paved the way for new 'penile preserving techniques' which minimised the impact of the disease and its treatment on quality of life, without compromising cancer control. A range of different techniques including topical chemotherapy, laser and reconstructive surgery are used, and tailored according to the stage, grade, and extent of disease (see Tables 16.1 and 16.2). In the UK, approximately 85% of new tumours are amenable to penis preserving treatments (see Figure 16.2).

Lymph node staging and treatment

Lymph nodes require surgical staging and are managed according to whether they are palpable at presentation (see Figure 16.3). Impalpable nodes harbour cancer in ~20%, while 50% of palpable nodes are cancerous. Impalpable nodes are best managed with dynamic sentinel lymph node biopsy (DSLNB), based on the predictable 'stepwise' spread of penile cancer from inguinal nodes, to pelvic nodes before any distant metastases develop. It detects the first draining 'sentinel' inguinal node after injection of a radio-labelled tracer around the primary tumour and has excellent sensitivity (95%) and a low complication rate (6%).

Table 16.1 2009 TNM classification of penile cancer.

Stage	Definition
Tis	Carcinoma in situ
Ta	Non-invasive verrucous carcinoma
T1a	Into sub-epithelial connective tissue: no high risk features
T1b	Into sub-epithelial connective tissue: high risk features
T2	Tumour invades corpus spongiosum/corpora cavernosum
T3	Tumour invades urethra
T4	Tumour invades other adjacent structures
pN0	No inguinal lymph nodes
pN1	Single inguinal lymph node metastasis
pN2	>1 inguinal lymph node metastasis
pN3	Fixed inguinal lymph node mass with extra-nodal spread, or metastasis in pelvic (iliac) lymph nodes
M1	Distant metastases

Table 16.2 Treatment options by stage.

Stage	Tis	Ta–T1a	T1b–T2	T3/T4
Treatment	Topical chemotherapy/ Immunotherapy (imiquimod, 5-fluorouracil)	*Foreskin* Circumcision	Glansectomy and reconstruction if no corpus cavernosum involvement Partial penectomy if corpus cavernosum involved or patient not fit for reconstruction	Partial penectomy for distal T3 Radical penectomy and perineal urethrostomy for proximal T2, high grade T3, any T4
	Laser (CO_2 or Nd:YAG) Glans resurfacing	*Glans* Wide local excision Glans resurfacing Glansectomy	Radiotherapy (if <4 cm)	+/− Chemo/Radiotherapy for advanced T4

(*Source:* TNM Classification 2009)

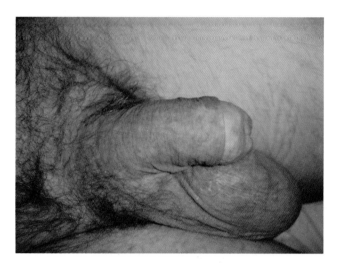

Figure 16.2 Glansectomy for distal penile cancer and reconstruction using split skin graft to create a near normal looking penis, with normal urinary and sexual function 6 months after surgery.

Role of chemotherapy and radiotherapy

The role of chemotherapy and the optimal regime remain unclear in penile cancer. It is used as:

1 Neo-adjuvant therapy to render inoperable cases operable
2 Adjuvant treatment for high risk disease with evidence of nodal spread
3 Palliative treatment for aggressive, metastatic disease in patients with good performance status.

Chemotherapy should only be used in a clinical trial setting to clarify its role and potential benefit.

Adjuvant radiotherapy is often used to improve local disease control in patients with extensive metastases or extra-nodal spread.

Follow-up

Local recurrence rates after penile preserving techniques can be as high as 30%. Most occur in the first two years. Early detection allows

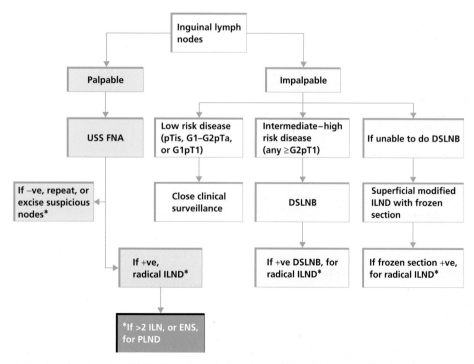

Figure 16.3 Management of regional lymph nodes. DSLNB: Dynamic sentinel lymph node biopsy, ILND: Inguinal lymph node dissection, ENS: Extra-nodal spread, PLND: Pelvic lymph node dissection, USS FNA: Ultrasound and fine needle aspiration cytology, ILN: Inguinal lymph nodes.

further penile preserving surgery, without any adverse oncological outcome. Patients are closely followed up 3-monthly for the first two years, reducing to 6-monthly to complete five years. After radical surgery the risk of recurrence is very low, and patients are seen 6-monthly for the first two years, reducing to annual visits up to five years.

Gender reassignment

Gender identity disorder (GID) (or gender dysphoria or transsexualism) is the strong identification of self with the opposite gender combined with significant social and mental distress from trying to function in the perceived wrong gender, in the absence of genetic or intersex anomalies. This may be difficult to distinguish from other conditions, so if suspected, patients must be referred to a specialist Gender Identity Clinic (GIC) for assessment (Box 16.3). Often GID is already established from the age of 2–4 years.

Box 16.3 Gender Identity Clinic – sequence of events

1 Assessment and Diagnosis
2 Psychotherapy
3 Real life experience (RLE)
4 Hormonal therapy
5 Sex reassignment surgery (SRS)

Real life experience (RLE)

Patients have to successfully dress and live in the chosen gender, preferably with a job or in education and provide evidence that at least one person outside the GIC accepts them in their chosen gender role.

Hormone therapy

The GIC will write to the patient's general practitioner to start oestrogen for MTF patients and testosterone for FTM patients. In the UK this is only legal once the patient is 18 years old. This is a stressful time for patients with major changes mentally and physically (Table 16.3 and Box 16.4). MTF patients may also get referred for speech therapy.

Box 16.4 Effects of oestrogen over 1–2 years

- Softer skin/hair
- Testis atrophy
- Erectile dysfunction
- Breast/nipple growth
- Reduced muscle mass
- Female fat distribution
- Reduced libido

Table 16.3 Effects of testosterone.

Immediate 3–6 months	Delayed up to 5 years
Periods stop	Laryngeal growth
Acne	Enlarged clitoris
Voice breaks	Increased muscle mass
Hair growth	Coarse skin
Increased libido	Less emotional
Increased appetite	Polycythaemia
	Male pattern baldness

Table 16.4 Sex reassignment surgery.

For MTF	For FTM
• Hair removal	• Mastectomy
• Tracheal shave	• Hysterectomy
• Facial reconstruction	• Oophorectomy
• Breast augmentation	• Vaginectomy
• Orchidectomy	• Urethroplasty
• Penectomy	• Metoidioplasty
• Vaginoplasty	• Phalloplasty

Sex reassignment surgery (SRS)

This is usually divided into top half and bottom half surgery with the genital surgery usually performed last (Table 16.4). The aim is for minimal donor site morbidity and scarring. This is far easier for MTF as compared to FTM patients. Removal of the gonads reduces the exogenous hormone requirement. More than 90% of transsexual patients are satisfied with the functional and cosmetic aspects of their SRS.

SRS for MTF

Facial hair removal is essential. The 'Adam's apple' is reduced by nibbling away at the tracheal cartilages to give a softer outline. The chin can be reshaped to be less square. A brow-lift will tidy up the forehead and age lines. If hormone induced breast enlargement is insufficient then a breast augmentation is performed. Orchidectomy is usually deferred until the time of vaginoplasty. The most common technique is a peno-scrotal inversion vaginoplasty.

SRS for FTM

The breast tissue is removed and the nipples and areola reduced and resited to a male anatomical position. A laparoscopic technique is preferred for hysterectomy and bilateral oophorectomy. Vaginectomy is not routine but can be requested for a more male appearance.

Phalloplasty (Figure 16.4)

This is the most difficult operation in SRS and is usually a multistage procedure. Patients have different requirements e.g. standing to void, pants filler, penetrative sex, phallus sensation. These requirements will dictate the type of surgery performed.

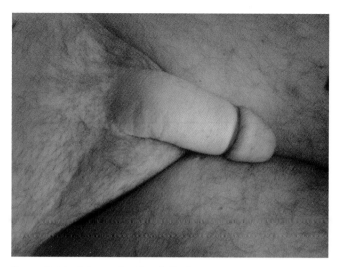

Figure 16.4 Radial artery free flap phalloplasty with glans sculpting and built in urethra but no erectile device.

Common long-term problems

Osteoporosis can occur with inadequate hormone therapy. Urethral stricture happens in both groups and can be difficult to treat. Smoking is discouraged for MTF because of the increased thrombogenic effect with oestrogens and for FTM patients because it increases the phalloplasty loss rate and long-term urethral stricture rate from ischaemia.

Further reading

Pizzocaro G, Algaba F, Horenblas S et al. EAU Penile cancer guidelines 2009. *Eur Urol* 2010: 57: 1002–12.

The Harry Benjamin International Gender Dysphoria Association's Standards of Care for Gender Identity Disorders, Sixth Version, February, 2001. From the World Professional Association for Transgender Health at http://www.wpath.org/.

Index